Down With Acid

(A book about Acid Reflux – its complications and management)

Copyright © Chris Robinson 2015

Published by The Sarsen Press, 22 Hyde Street, Winchester, Hampshire, SO23 7DR

First Edition April 2016

Second (revised) Edition July 2017

PREFACE

Concerns about acid reflux can range from occasional indigestion after a large meal, to life threatening diseases such as cancer. This book is designed as a reference to help sufferers whatever stage their problem is.

Symptoms of acid reflux: Although there are many symptoms that could be attributable to acid reflux, from severe abdominal cramps to dry eyes, from vomiting blood to dizziness, many may not experience any identifiable symptoms at all. It is also important to remember that many of the symptoms listed may be attributable to other factors which may need to be ruled out first.

The most commonly identified symptom is heartburn (which is nothing to do with the heart).
Chest pains may be from acid reflux but an ECG may be necessary to determine they aren't actually from the heart.
"Water Brash" is an excess of saliva or a bitter taste to the saliva that may be an indication of acid (or bile) reflux.
Difficulty swallowing should always be investigated by a doctor.

An extensive list of other possible symptoms may be found in the chapter on Extra-Oesophageal Reflux or see the symptom checker in the appendix.

FOREWORDS

About the author

After 30 years as a teacher, deputy head and adviser for science and technology for 4-13 year olds, Chris took early retirement on health grounds and now spends time working for Barrett's Wessex, the charity he co-founded. He is a previous trustee of the charity, Barrett's Oesophagus Campaign (BOC), and a committee member of Action Against Heartburn (AAH).

He is a keen cyclist and has cycled to raise funds in Europe, East Asia and South America.

You may read a summary of Chris's Story in the Appendix.

About Barrett's Wessex charity

In 1999, BOC was founded to maintain the UK Barrett's Oesophagus Registry (UKBOR), with a patient support arm including an on-line forum.

Shortly after he discovered the forum in 2008, Chris responded to a post, "Southampton anyone?" wherein a patient suggested it could be beneficial to meet up with others to discuss their condition. A year later the "Barrett's Support Network – Wessex area" group was formed following an inaugural meeting attended by over 100 people.

After raising funds to purchase a Radio Frequency Ablation machine for Southampton hospital, the group became an independent charity, "Barrett's Wessex", to enable them to concentrate on patients' needs leaving BOC to concentrate on UKBOR, an invaluable resource to researchers.

About the same time, BOC and another charity, Oesophageal Patients Association (OPA) co-founded AAH, now a consortium of all UK charities concerned with raising awareness of oesophageal cancer. AAH campaigned to get the NHS to run a Be Clear On Cancer campaign on oesophago-gastric cancers in 2015.

Author's notes

Acid reflux and its complications is one of the most common complaints in the Western world and there are many charlatans and snake oil salesmen ready to exploit the misery of the gullible and desperate unwary. "Barrett's Esophagus Cure" says the headline while the small print asks $29.95 to let you download the misguided and potentially harmful file.

This book is largely composed of answers provided at various times to questions posed on on-line forums. Apologies if there are some duplications of information. It is intended to be an encyclopaedia to be dipped into as required.

I have attempted to tear a hole in a shroud to reveal detail beneath. As with all holes, there'll be some loose threads which could be unravelled making the hole bigger but leaving even more loose threads.

I am not a doctor but can speak on most of the contents of this book from first hand experience and from the experiences of the hundreds I have met either in person or in on-line forums and facebook pages. - *This book should not replace any advice provided by your GP.*

Copyright

This book is freely downloadable from www.DownWithAcid.org.uk by anyone who will find it helpful. It may be distributed freely (as long as it is kept intact and not edited - including cover pages). It cannot be sold for personal gain. Printed copies may be made available at a cost to cover materials and if any profits are made or donations received, they should be forwarded to Barrett's Wessex.

Acknowlegements

Illustrations

Although some illustrations are the creation of the author, most are believed to be public domain or the creator's consent has been received.

Inclusion within this work of illustrations from commercial medical companies does not imply their endorsement of this work nor vice versa.

Apologies are offered if inadvertently copyright has been breached. If you believe this to be so, please inform the author immediately so this may be addressed.

Accuracy and proof-reading

The author would like to thank all the specialist medics, surgeons and nurses for taking the time to check the accuracy of this work and the patients who have checked for legibility.

Language

Whereas this book is primarily in UK English, some American spellings may be encountered, particularly in quotations from research papers where US English was originally used. These include esophagus for oesophagus and GERD for GORD.

Contents

	Page
Introduction	
Digestive System, Indigestion, Heartburn, GORD	3
Acid	
Too much, Too little	7
Medicines	8
Natural remedies	11
Bile	
Gallstones, Cholestrerol	19
Reflux	
Hiatus Hernia, Heartburn, GORD	23
Extra-Oesophageal Reflux (LPR / "Silent" reflux)	24
Natural Remedies	26
Reflux reduction techniques - medication, surgery and devices	
Fundoplication (various)	29
LINX	32
Stretta	33
Esophyx (TIF), MUSE, Endocinch	34
Endostim	38
Enteryx, Gatekeeper	39
Angelchik	40
Reza Band	41
MedCline	42
Food	
Acid and Alkaline Foods	48
Foods that may cause Reflux	48
Know your triggers	48
Some Food Myths	49
How we eat is important	50
Exercise after food	50

Combinations and Complications

Oesophagitis	**53**
Barrett's Oesophagus	**54**
Put Simply	**56**
Oesophageal Cancer	**57**
Swallowing difficulties: strictures, achalasia, dysphagia	**59**
Nutcracker oesophagus	**60**
Induced Hypochlorhydria	**60**
Small Intestinal Fungal / Bacterial Overgrowth (SIFO /SIBO)	**61**

Tests and Diagnosis:

Self Diagnosis	**65**
Endoscopy	**66**
Biopsies	**67**
Cytosponge	**69**
Peptest	**70**
24 hr pH manometry, Bravo 48 hour monitoring, DeMeester score	**71**
Barium swallow, Heidelberg test	**72**

Treatments

Recommendations	**74**
Endoscopic Mucosal Resection	**76**
Radio Frequency Ablation	**76**
Cryotherapy	**77**
Photo Dynamic Therapy	**78**
Argon Plasma Coagulation	**78**
Oesophagectomy	**79**

Other related conditions / complications, side effects etc

Otorhinolaryngological (ENT)	**83**
Pneumonia	**84**
Chronic Obstructive Pulmonary Disease (COPD)	**84**
Bronchiectasis	**85**
Pulmonary Fibrosis (IPF)	**85**
Gastric Dumping Syndrome	**86**
Eosinophilic Oesophagitis (EoE)	**87**

Myths and Misconceptions
    False Profits, Acid & Alkaline foods, Cancer myths   **91**

Appendices
    Symptom checker   **95**
    NICE Option Grid for treatment of long term heartburn   **96**
    Help – where to find more information and get support   **97**
    Author's experiences   **99**

References
    101

Introduction

Understanding the digestive system.

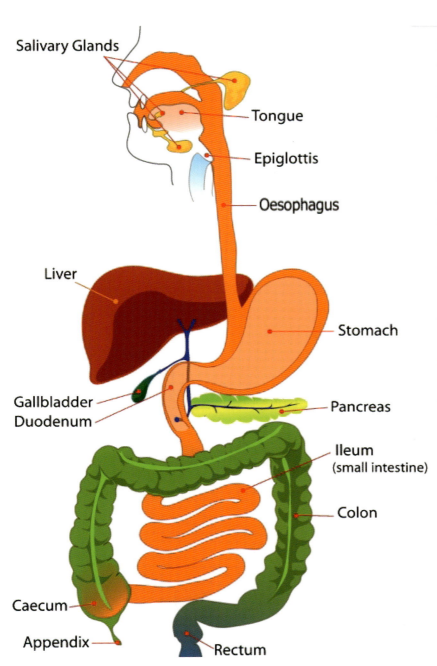

The first stage of digestion is chewing involving teeth and saliva to make small enough pieces to swallow.
At the back of the throat, the epiglottis closes over the trachea (windpipe) so the food bolus enters the oesophagus, the food tube that passes through the chest to the stomach, instead of the lungs.

Along the length of the oesophagus, muscles squeeze the tube above the bolus to push it towards the stomach. This is called peristalsis.

In the stomach, the bolus is churned in concentrated acid to liquidise it into chyme which can pass out of the stomach into the duodenum where it meets bile and digestive enzymes to enable absorption to continue along the intestines.

There are various rings of muscles along the way to act as valves as the whole tract is intended to be a one way street. These are called sphincters.

At the top of the oesophagus, the upper oesophageal sphincter is composed mainly of the cricopharyngeus to permit food to remain in the oesophagus rather than the airways.

At the base of the oesophagus, the lower oesophageal sphincter is joined with muscles of the diaphragm to permit matter to enter the stomach and keep it there.

If any matter flows the wrong way through any of these sphincters, it's called reflux.

Indigestion may refer to any abnormality within the digestive process.

One of the most commonly reported is **heartburn** which has nothing to do with the heart but is actually acid attacking the oesophagus when stomach acid refluxes via the lower oesophageal sphincter.

Gastro-Oesophageal Reflux Disorder (or Disease) "**GORD**" describes the condition where heartburn occurs frequently, although not everyone who has GORD experiences the pain of heartburn.

The Oesophagus

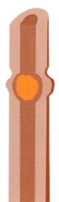

Muscles above the food bolus contract while muscles below relax to help propel the food along the oesophagus.

This is a tube about 25 cm long and 2 cm wide when inactive. I liken it to a bicycle tyre inner tube.

The walls of the oesophagus comprise, from inside outwards, the mucosa, the submucosa, the muscularis propria (musculature for peristalsis) and the adventia (the outer wall).

The mucosa produces mucous to lubricate and protect the oesopagus.

The stomach

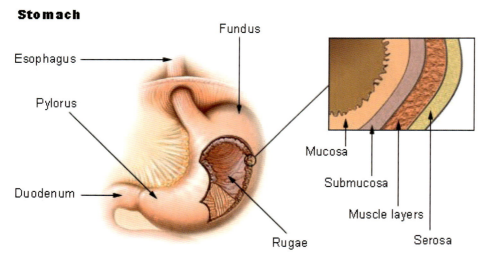

In its mucosa, triggered by the ingestion of food, the stomach produces proton pumps, special cells that, by releasing protons into the gastric juices, render it highly acidic making concentrated hydrochloric acid with a pH typically of 1.

Section 1 – Acid

Medication

There are 4 major classes of drugs to treat the acid element of acid reflux. In ascending order of effectiveness, they are antacids, alginates, H2 blockers and Proton Pump Inhibitors.

If you need to use any of these drugs frequently, please seek medical advice.

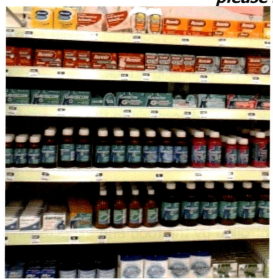

1. Antacids

They work immediately on excess acid. They do not prevent excess acid occurring.

These are drugs that neutralise the acid. Most commonly they are made of chalk, calcium carbonate. Examples are Tums or Rennie. Chemically, this reaction takes place:

$$CaCO_3 + 2HCl \rightarrow CaCl_2 + H_2O + CO_2$$

(Calcium Carbonate + Hydrochloric acid gives Calcium Chloride (a harmless salt) plus water and carbon dioxide).

2. Alginates

Gaviscon is the brand name of the white milky liquid that floats on the stomach contents as oil floats on water to reduce the possibility of reflux whilst also providing a temporary protective film to the lower oesophagus and neutralising the acid with an antacid component. (Some generic versions are now available.)

	NHS cost for 28 days
Gaviscon	£5.84

3. H2 blockers

Histamine H2 Receptor Antagonists work to block the histamine signals that tell the stomach to produce acid. (N.B. This is not the same as an antihistamine.)

The most common is Ranitidine, brand name Zantac but others are available as shown below.

These work proactively to reduce the amount of acid rather than being an instant antacid. Often prescribed to be taken in the evening to reduce night time reflux of acid.

Generic name	Brand name	Dose *	NHS cost for 28 days (2011)
Ranitidine	Zantac	150 mg 300 mg	£1.35 £1.28
Famotidine	Pepsid	40 mg	£4.68
Cimetidine	Tagamet	400 mg	£6.27
Nizatidine	Axid	300 mg	£9.81

(Other H2 blockers: Lafutidine, Loxtidine, Niperotidine, Roxatidine.)

Section 1 – Acid

ACID

Acid is needed by the body but too much or too little or in the wrong place can cause problems.

Hydrochloric acid is produced by the stomach to aid digestion and combat harmful bacteria. It should remain in the stomach and the quantity and strength varies depending upon need.

This acid is dangerous stuff: it's strong enough to dissolve metal. If you were to spill it on your skin, it would burn and cause scarring. The stomach is protected by being lined with special cells that constantly produce a layer of mucous to prevent acid attack.

The acid helps turn the food bolus entering the stomach from the oesophagus into liquid chyme and leaches essential minerals from the food for better absorption in the intestines.

Oils and fats, however, do not mix with the acid and if they need to be broken down some bile may need to be released into the stomach via the pylorus. [a-i]

Another important role of the acid is in protection against disease as it can kill harmful ingested bacteria.

The amount and strength of acid in the stomach is controlled by the food and expectation of it through hormonal signals from the thyroid gland. The production of acid also triggers production of pepsin and other enzymes which help break down proteins.

If the stomach produces **too much acid** (hyperchlorhydria), the mucous may be insufficient to protect the stomach lining. Inflammation (gastritis) or ulcers can form.

Whether stress can cause too much acid is a matter of debate. Anecdotally, many who suffer with excess stomach acid report it having been exacerbated by stress which could be due to reduced levels of a protein called TFF2 which helps repair acid damage. [a-ii]

Too little stomach acid (hypochlorhydria) can result in poor absorption of essential elements and reduced bacterial immunity.

Many people have the bacteria **H-Pylori** (helicobacter-pylori) living in their gut. For some people this can be the cause of stomach ulcers. They do not like an acid environment and burrow deep into the stomach walls where acid levels are more neutral. [a-iii]

Presence of H-Pylori is detected with a breath test, a blood test, a stool test or a biopsy.

H-Pylori is treated with a mixture of antibiotics.

Keeping it in its place.

From the stomach, the liquid chyme flows out through the pyloric sphincter into the duodenum and intestines. It may still be acidic though may be partially neutralised by the bile it encounters in the duodenum. The columnar structure of the cells lining the intestines, along with more mucous, makes them resistant to acid.

The top of the stomach is held shut by muscles collectively known as the Lower Oesophageal Sphincter to prevent the possibility of the acid splashing back into the oesophagus.

Medication

There are 4 major classes of drugs to treat the acid element of acid reflux. In ascending order of effectiveness, they are antacids, alginates, H2 blockers and Proton Pump Inhibitors.

***If you need to use any of these drugs frequently,
please seek medical advice.***

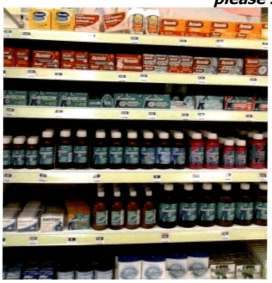

1. Antacids

They work immediately on excess acid. They do not prevent excess acid occurring.
These are drugs that neutralise the acid. Most commonly they are made of chalk, calcium carbonate. Examples are Tums or Rennie. Chemically, this reaction takes place:
$$CaCO_3 + 2HCl \rightarrow CaCl_2 + H_2O + CO_2$$
(Calcium Carbonate + Hydrochloric acid gives Calcium Chloride (a harmless salt) plus water and carbon dioxide).

2. Alginates

Gaviscon is the brand name of the white milky liquid that floats on the stomach contents as oil floats on water to reduce the possibility of reflux whilst also providing a temporary protective film to the lower oesophagus and neutralising the acid with an antacid component. (Some generic versions are now available.)

	NHS cost for 28 days
Gaviscon	£5.84

3. H2 blockers

Histamine H2 Receptor Antagonists work to block the histamine signals that tell the stomach to produce acid. (N.B. This is not the same as an antihistamine.)
The most common is Ranitidine, brand name Zantac but others are available as shown below.

These work proactively to reduce the amount of acid rather than being an instant antacid. Often prescribed to be taken in the evening to reduce night time reflux of acid.

Generic name	Brand name	Dose *	NHS cost for 28 days (2011)
Ranitidine	Zantac	150 mg 300 mg	£1.35 £1.28
Famotidine	Pepsid	40 mg	£4.68
Cimetidine	Tagamet	400 mg	£6.27
Nizatidine	Axid	300 mg	£9.81

(Other H2 blockers: Lafutidine, Loxtidine, Niperotidine, Roxatidine.)

* Please note doses shown are not guaranteed to be equivalent. Do not assume because a dose is shown it is the safe dose. It may vary according to age and body build.

4. Proton Pump Inhibitors (PPIs)

These are the most effective drugs to reduce acid production. They work by effectively stopping the creation of some of the cells (proton pumps) that produce acid in the stomach.

There are a number known by different names as shown in the table below. The equivalent dose shown is the "maintenance dose" though you may be prescribed a higher dose initially. They are proactive drugs and are most effective after taking them for a few days. They do not neutralise acid already produced.

Generic name	UK brand name	US brand name	Equivalent dose *(approx)*	NHS cost for 28 days (2011)
Omeprazole	Losec	Prilosec	20 mg	£1.68
Lansoprazole	Zoton	Prevacid	30 mg	£2.08
Pantoprazole	Protium	Protonix	40 mg	£16.43
Rabeprazole	Pariet	Aciphex	20 mg	£19.55
Esomeprazole	Nexium	Nexium	20 mg 40mg *	£18.50 £25.19
Dexlansoprazole	Dexilant	Kapidex / Dexilant	30 mg	N/A

(Other PPIs: Ilaprazole, Picoprazole, Tenatoprazole, Timoprazole)

Do not assume because a dose is shown it is the safe dose. It may vary according to age and body build.

The most common brand names are shown though they may also be known under other names in other parts of the world.

Research evidence has shown all PPIs are as effective as each other (though the drugs companies may try to make us believe otherwise) but some may be better tolerated by some patients. [a-iv][a-v]

* Astra Zeneca (who make the drug) claims 40mg esomeprazole is equivalent to 20mg omeprazole and one (Astra Zeneca sponsored) trial showed 40mg esomeprazole was better at reducing acid production than 20mg omeprazole. [a-vi]
Another study published February 2015 [a-vii] also compared 40mg esomeprazole with 30mg lansoprazole and 40mg Pantoprazole finding: "esomeprazole was more effective".

Research funded by Reckitt Benkiser (who make the drug) found Gaviscon was no less effective than standard dose omeprazole for a 24hr period. [a-viii]

Controversy over long term medication

The efficacy of long term use of acid suppressant medication (particularly PPIs) has been questioned with some claiming they cause oesteoporosis, hypermagnesaemia, and even cancer. Whereas these claims are not entirely unfounded, the evidence is disputed. See "hypochlorhydria" (pg 60) and "Myths and Misconceptions" (pg 91).

PPIs have been linked to Myocardial Infarction [a-ix]. That those with heart conditions may be greater amongst those taking PPIs is not surprising since the symptoms of heart attack and indigestion can be so similar. The "evidence" shows a correlation not a causation.

A more recent study [a-x] followed 54,422 GERD patients in Taiwan compared with 269,572 randomly selected age-, gender-, comorbidity-matched subjects, finding, amongst other things, "patients who were prescribed PPIs for more than one year had slightly decreased the risk of developing Acute Myocardial Infarction".

Similarly PPIs have been associated with Chronic Kidney Disease [a-xi]. Again this showed a correlation: those with kidney problems are more likely to be users of PPIs.

Another study looking at the medicines used by patients over the age of 75 with dementia, found a higher proportion of them used PPIs than amongst the general population. [a-xii] Another case of correlation rather than causation and some doctors were led to speak out about misinterpreting the data. [a-xiii.]

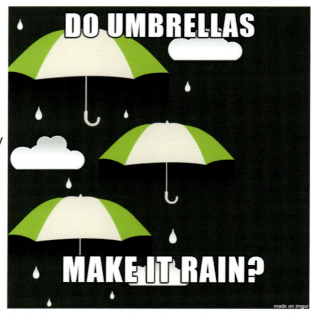

A paper published in Gastroenterology in June 2017 [a-xiv], however, found no association between the use of proton pump inhibitors and the risk for mild cognitive impairment, dementia and Alzheimer's disease

Another paper published in 2013 appeared to show PPIs could cause oesophageal cancer [a-xv].
This quickly received rebuffs: [a-xvi.]

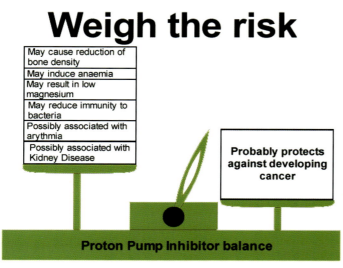

The popular media loves scare stories like these and, never letting the facts get in the way of a good story, can exaggerate them causing real fear amongst some PPI users who often try turning to unproven "natural" remedies for their condition that may do more harm than good.

A Danish study in 2014 had concluded: "No cancer-protective effects from PPI's were seen. In fact, high-adherence and long-term use of PPI were associated with a significantly increased risk of adenocarcinoma or high-grade dysplasia." [a-xvii] in contradiction of a 2013 study which concluded: "The use of PPIs is associated with a decreased risk of OAC and/or BO-HGD in patients with BO. None of the studies showed an increased risk of OAC." [a-xviii] and an article published in 2014 which claimed a protective effect for PPIs. [a-xix]

There has been research however that shows PPIs most probably have a chemo-protective effect helping reduce incidences of oesophageal cancer as published in a 2014 meta-analysis [a-xx] finding "PPI use was associated with a 71% reduction in risk of OAC and/or BO-HGD in patients with BO."

Another paper, "PPIs display antitumor effects in Barrett's adenocarcinoma [a-xxi]" also found "evidence supporting the potential use of PPIs as novel antineoplastic drugs for EAC".

The 2014 NICE guidelines on the management of GORD [a-xxii] made the recommendation to Consider laparoscopic fundoplication for people who have:

- a confirmed diagnosis of acid reflux and adequate symptom control with acid suppression therapy, but who do not wish to continue with this therapy long term

- a confirmed diagnosis of acid reflux and symptoms that are responding to a PPI, but who cannot tolerate acid suppression therapy.

An Option Grid produced by NICE may be found in the Appendices.

"Natural" remedies

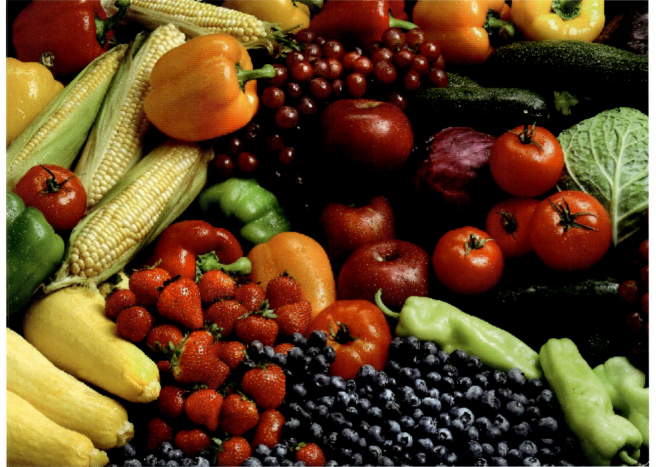

Most fruits and vegetables may have beneficial properties for acid reflux sufferers.

This chapter includes complementary and alternative treatments some claim can help treat excess acid. Research evidence seems to be lacking in the great majority of cases so claims presented here are mainly anecdotal.

The long list presented includes treatments which some people have found useful. They are not provided as recommendations but for information only. If you wish to try any of them, you do so in this knowledge.

Whilst complementary treatments may be beneficial for some in reducing some symptoms, it is not recommended they are used as an alternative to replace conventional treatment. Complementary treatments should always be notified and discussed with your doctor in case of harmful interactions with prescribed medication.

Chewing Gum

By chewing gum, more saliva is produced which may help neutralise excess acid.

Turmeric

The active component of Turmeric is curcumin. Currently there is no research evidence to show that turmeric or curcumin can prevent or treat cancer but early trials have shown some promising results.

A number of studies have shown curcumin can kill some cancer cells and prevent more from growing.

In an American study reported in 2008, "25 patients had curcumin treatment and 21 had tumours that could be measured. In 2 patients their tumours shrank or remained stable. In some patients their levels of particular immune system chemicals that destroy cancer cells went up. But the researchers found that blood levels of curcumin were very low because it is not well absorbed from the gut. Scientists have since developed injectable, fat soluble forms of curcumin which may improve the results." [r-xlvii]

Ginger

Some people swear by ginger root tea as a preparation for the stomach before food. It is made by steeping cut pieces of ginger root in simmering water for half an hour and proponents say to drink a cupful half an hour before you eat claiming it acts as some sort of buffer to acid production.

Aloe Vera

There are many claims made for aloe vera. It's main use as a balm is to soothe abrasions. This may explain its popularity for those with acid reflux or oesophagitis.

Cancer Research UK has carried out research into the healing properties of aloe and the claims made for it. They found there was no evidence to suggest that aloe vera works but many patients say that they have found aloe helpful. Some early research seems to suggest that it may help wounds to heal. Early studies of aloe substances in laboratory animals seem to suggest that some of the chemicals found in aloe may have helpful effects on the immune system and can shrink some cancers.

Some users of aloe may experience side effects of diarrhoea, nausea and stomach pain.

Aloe vera may interact with other drugs or herbs so always talk to your doctor before you begin taking it.

"Once people begin taking aloe supplements regularly, they tend to develop a tolerance, requiring increased doses to maintain the effect. As the dose increases, safety is of increasing concern: case reports of fatalities and severe kidney dysfunction have been reported with high doses." *[U.S.News - Health & Wellness]*

Slippery Elm

The active ingredient of slippery elm is a polysaccharide called mucilage that makes a slippery gel when wet.

As with aloe vera, slippery elm is a soothing balm and may help digestive motility by stimulating the secretion of mucous in the digestive tract.

It is not recommended in people who have kidney or liver problems the plants contain chemicals called oxalates which can damage the liver and kidneys.

Deglycerised Liquorice

As with aloe vera and slippery elm above, liquorice is a demulcent forming a soothing layer over inflammation and possibly increasing production of mucous thus providing symptom relief.

"However, while liqorice contains beneficial phytochemicals, it also contains glycyrrhizic acid, which is associated with side effects. To counter this, a modified form of the botanical medicine, known as deglycyrrhizinated licorice, or DGL licorice, is available. Although considered safer, DGL licorice may still pose certain health risks." [Livestrong]

Green Tea

"Green tea is a drink made from the dried leaves of the Asian plant Camellia sinensis. This tea is drunk widely across Asia. The rates of many cancers are much lower in Asia than other parts of the world. Some people believe this is because of the high intake of green tea. The substance in green tea that researchers think is most helpful is called epigallocatechin-3-gallate (EGCG). EGCG is available as green tea extract which some people take as a supplement in liquid or capsules." [Cancer Research UK]

"Fifty-one studies with more than 1.6 million participants, mainly of observational nature were included in this systematic review. Studies looked for an association between green tea consumption and cancer of the digestive tract, ... The evidence that the consumption of green tea might reduce the risk of cancer was conflicting. This means, that drinking green tea remains unproven in cancer prevention, but appears to be safe at moderate, regular and habitual use." [Cochrane review]

Apple Cider Vinegar

Proponents of apple cider vinegar suggest two to three teaspoonfuls should be stirred into a small glass of water to be consumed before every meal and offer two alternative theories as to why it may work.

1. By providing acid to the stomach before food, the stomach may be fooled into expecting more acid and therefore doesn't need to produce so much.

2. The Lower Oesophageal Sphincter muscles are activated to tighten by acid; drinking ACV before a meal "wakes up" the LOS.

Both of these claims, however, fail to recognise the comparative strengths of stomach acid, which can dissolve metal and would produce scarring if spilled on the skin, and ACV whose only effect on the skin would be to make it feel wet.

A paper "Is Apple Cider Vinegar Effective for Reducing Heartburn?" published in 2015 [a-xxiii] found, "compared to the placebo trial, the vinegar trials do not show significant alleviation of the heartburn sensation and an article published in "Foods 4 Better Heath" in February 2017 [a-xxiv] warned about side effects of drinking too much ACV.

Lemon Water

One recipe suggests: "To neutralize stomach acids, add more alkalinity to your stomach. Mix a squeeze of lemon (about 1-2 tsp) in a cup of warm water. This will raise your alkaline level." [Philippine Daily Enquirer magazine]

However there is no evidence to suggest or support the theory and no explanation is presented as to why acid lemon juice should increase alkalinity.

Mustard

Some claim that a teaspoon of made mustard eaten straight can help neutralise acid reflux if taken immediately it is noticed. Proponents assert it to be alkaline and thus neutralises stomach acid.

Manuka honey

There are a number of medicinal properties for honey, the main ones being its anti-bacterial and anti-inflammatory properties. Sterilised medical grade honey may be used as a wound dressing.

Honey is sometimes used in cough medication or for sore throats. Along with the properties noted above, it's texture and mucous inducing properties have a soothing influence.

However, research evidence that it may help with gastrointestinal problems is lacking.

Kombucha

Kombucha tea is brewed using kombucha which is a type of yeast, black tea and sugar. The resulting alcoholic vinegary drink has many health claims attributed to it. However none have been substantiated and no explanation has been provided why it should benefit acid reflux sufferers.

There have, however, been reports of adverse effects, such as stomach upset, infections and allergic reactions in kombucha tea drinkers.

The Mayo Clinic in America says "there isn't good evidence that kombucha tea delivers on its health claims. At the same time, several cases of harm have been reported. Therefore, the prudent approach is to avoid kombucha tea until more definitive information is available."

Peppermint

Peppermint is often used as an aid for digestion problems. "Peppermint water can relieve trapped wind and so relieve pain. Put a few drops of peppermint oil in hot water and sip it slowly." [Cancer Research UK]

Clinical trials have proved it beneficial for lower gastric tract problems such as irritable bowel.

However, it works by relaxing the pyloric sphincter muscles which helps the egress of bile to assist digestion and relieving pressure building up at the stomach exit. By relaxing the Lower Oesophageal Sphincter also, it helps release trapped gas from the stomach but also exacerbates gastro-oesophageal reflux so those with acid reflux should avoid it.

Marijuana

There have been many studies into the medicinal properties of cannabinoids (eg marijuana) with many on-going around the world presently. Beneficial properties are being found particularly in areas of pain relief. Like Peppermint, the benefits of the drug are as a muscle relaxant.

There are many claims made for benefits of the drug on gastric problems. MedicalMarijuana.com says,"Research suggests that cannabis is effective in treating the symptoms of these GI disorders in part because it interacts with the endogenous cannabinoid receptors in the digestive tract, which can result in calming spasms, assuaging pain, and improving motility. Cannabis has also been shown to have anti-inflammatory properties and recent research shows crucial neuromodulatory roles in controlling the operation of the gastrointestinal system, with synthetic and natural cannabinoids acting powerfully to control gastrointestinal motility and inflammation." but, although a list of references is published on the site, it hasn't been possible to find the paper this quotes.

The concern is, like Peppermint above, the "calming" and "improving motility" may also exacerbate reflux.

Cancer Research UK issue this advice: "Although centuries of human experimentation tells us that naturally-occurring cannabinoids are broadly safe, they are not without risks. They can increase the heart rate, which may cause problems for patients with pre-existing or undiagnosed heart conditions. They can also interact with other drugs in the body, including antidepressants and antihistamines. And they may also affect how the body processes certain chemotherapy drugs, which could cause serious side effects."

Baking Soda

This age old remedy is the basis of most antacids like Tums or Rennie which are immediate acting by neutralising the stomach acid. Baking Soda is the chemical Sodium Bicarbonate, $NaHCO_3$. (Antacids may use other similar compounds such as calcium carbonate or magnesium carbonate but they have a similar effect.)

Chemically, this reaction takes place:

$$NaHCO_3 + HCl \rightarrow NaCl + H_2O + CO_2$$

(Sodium Bicarbonate + Hydrochloric acid gives Sodium Chloride (table salt) plus water and carbon dioxide)   *Compare "Antacids" page 8*

Almonds

It has been suggested that 3 or 4 almonds eaten after a meal may help prevent reflux.

N.B. Some may experience an adverse reaction to almonds which can produce migraine attacks in some people.

Apples, Bananas

Eating an apple or a banana a day are also suggested. Many fruits have been shown to be beneficial to health.

Books on how to cure your acid reflux may be found being sold as downloads on the internet extolling the values of different fruits for curing acid reflux. Most of these appear to exist primarily as a source of income for their authors who usually have no medical qualification.

Japanese Apricot

Japanese Apricot has recently been found to be a possible aid to motility. In 2010, GORD-related symptoms were examined in 1303 Japanese individuals using a validated questionnaire. Those who consumed Japanese Apricot daily (either dried or pickled) showed significantly improved scores compared with subjects who did not. [r-xlviii]

Section 2 – Bile

BILE

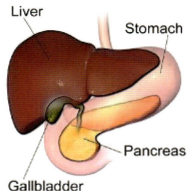

Bile is a bitter tasting green liquid made by the liver and stored in the gall bladder. Its principal job is to help the absorption and dispersal of fats. Acting like detergent, it permits the emulsification of fats and water – like washing up liquid on a greasy plate.

As the liquid chyme passes out of the stomach, large amounts of bile are released from the gall bladder into the duodenum. If fats remain in the stomach too long, some bile may be permitted to back flow through the pyloric sphincter to help. [a-i]

Bile is produced by the liver and stored in the gall bladder. Along with enzymes produced by the pancreas, bile passes into the duodenum via the hepatopancreatic sphincter, usually referred to as the sphincter of Oddi. If required in the stomach, it is permitted to backflow through the pylorus, the normal exit route from the stomach.

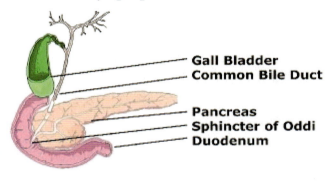

Vitamins A, D, E and K are all fat soluble and require the action of bile to be absorbed into the body.

Bile also helps in the transport of waste materials, including those filtered out in the liver, from the body and helps remove harmful bacteria from the body. The bile salts used in this transport system are reabsorbed into the blood stream at the end of the intestinal tract and returned to the liver for recycling.

Too much bile can cause diarrhoea. [b-i] Too little bile can result in malabsorption of essential vitamins, a build up of toxins in the liver and excess acid problems through inadequate neutralisation of it. Bloating after food may be a symptom of insufficient bile.

It has been suggested that reduced stomach acid resulting in poor initial breakdown of foodstuffs in the stomach, may trigger production of more bile to travel to the stomach to assist or, conversely, may mean less bile is required leading to a build up of bile in the gallbladder. Whatever the reason, those coping with stomach acid problems, seem to be more likely to experience problems with their gall bladder.

GALLSTONES

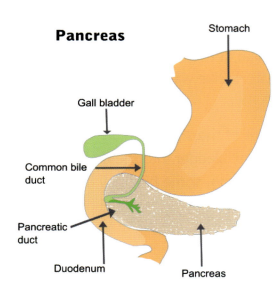

The gall bladder is the reservoir where bile produced by the liver is stored.

Gallstones and cholecystitis (inflammation of the gall bladder often caused by gallstones) have often been found to occur in patients with acid reflux. Whether one causes the other or both share a common cause isn't clear with research papers contradicting each other.

A paper published in 1936 in the Annals of Surgery reported a correlation between acute cholecystitis and reflux [b-ii] though a 2001 paper published in the American Journal of gastroenterology found no association between gallstones and gastroesophageal reflux disease [b-iii].

Gallstones are hard deposits which can form in this bladder. Frequently they cause no problem but sometimes may result in considerable pain. It may not be clear what causes gallstones: they are composed of "biliary sludge" that usually contains cholesterol.

It is suggested some "cholesterol reducing" drugs can result in a build up of cholesterol in bile. Other suggestions are the gall bladder isn't emptying efficiently or frequently enough or the liver may excrete an excess of cholesterol to the gall bladder.

Cholesterol

Cholesterol is an essential component of cell walls. it is also used by the liver to make bile, it makes Vitamin D and adrenal and sex hormones. It is transported around the body in the bloodstream by lipoproteins which come in two sorts, Low Density Lipoproteins (LDL, when we call it "bad cholesterol") and High Density Lipoproteins (HDL, when we call it "good cholesterol"). It's the LDL which can cause arteries to block up leading to heart attacks.

Section 3 – Reflux

Reflux

Reflux means a backflow of liquid in the body. Most commonly it is used for the backflow of contents from the stomach into the oesophagus, usually occasioned by a weak or malfunctioning Lower Oesophageal Sphincter (LOS). This is known as Gastro-Oesophageal Reflux (GOR) and if it persists it is called Gastro-Oesophageal Reflux Disorder (or Disease) - GORD for short.

Gastro-oesophageal reflux

The LOS works with the muscles of the crural diaphragm (at the base of the ribcage and used in breathing) to hold the oesophagus shut most of the time. However, when our bodies are in an upright position, occasional transient relaxation of the muscles is permitted to release gas - as a burp or belch.

For many people, the Lower Oesophageal Sphincter doesn't work as well as it should permitting stomach contents to flow back into the oesophagus.

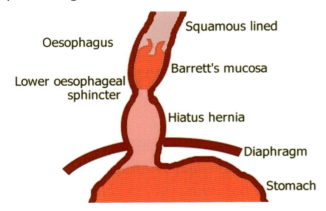

One of the most common reasons for this is a **hiatus hernia**. The hiatus is the hole in the diaphragm the oesophagus passes through just above its junction with the stomach. In many people, the top of the stomach can push up through this hole. Known as a hiatus hernia, we don't always know why this happens. Some people may have been born with a larger hiatus enabling herniation to occur at a young age. For others, the upward pressure caused by excess body fat may be the contributing factor.

For most people a hiatus hernia will cause no problems but for others, their sphincter muscles may not be strong enough to keep the end of the oesophagus tightly closed.

Excess body weight and abdominal fat can put pressure on the stomach pushing the contents back up the oesophagus, but even fit, normal weight people can experience reflux. Amongst other causes may be tight clothing, vigorous exercise after food or simply bending over. If the LOS isn't functioning properly, stomach contents may be forced back through it.

Heartburn is the symptom most commonly associated with acid reflux but 30% of those with acid reflux report not having experienced it for some reason. The pain is from the acid attacking the top layer of the oesophagus. It may be those who don't experience the pain are less susceptible to pain, the mucous dilutes the acid sufficiently for it not to burn or their cells may have become desensitised by transformation (e.g. from squamous to columnar as occurs with Barrett's Oesophagus). Prolonged acid attack can cause scarring and inflammation called oesophagitis.

The term **Gastro-Oesophageal Reflux Disease** (GORD) may be used when someone experiences reflux symptoms frequently.

The term, **Non-Erosive Reflux Disorder** (NERD) may be used when someone has GORD but without acid.

If GOR occurs, material may continue to the top of the oesophagus where it joins the trachea at the back of the throat. There is a weak flap valve here that is normally closed over the entrance of the oesophagus to allow respiration to occur. It automatically opens when swallowing to permit food to pass into the oesophagus rather than the lungs. It is controlled by the cricopharyngeal muscle. Although it may spasm, giving a "lump in the throat" feeling (called **globus**), it isn't very effective at stopping reflux which can aspirate throughout the respiratory system.

Extra-Oesophageal Reflux / LaryngoPharyngeal Reflux / Silent reflux

If reflux persists, it can traverse the entire column of the oesophagus and breach the upper oesophageal sphincter, a group of muscles including the cricopharyngeus that open when swallowing to permit food to enter the oesophagus rather than the trachea (windpipe).

Reflux occurring here is correctly termed extra-oesophageal reflux but is often referred to as "Laryngo-Pharyngeal Reflux" (LPR for short), "Respiratory Reflux" or "Silent Reflux". (The term 'silent reflux' is also often applied to lower oesophageal reflux where heartburn is not experienced.)

Even if the acid has been reduced or neutralised with acid suppressants or antacids, regurgitation of stomach contents and extra-oesophageal reflux (known as Non-Erosive Reflux Disorder, or NERD) can still cause damage.

From the top of the oesophagus it enters the respiratory system where it can aspirate into the throat, lungs, mouth and nose.

Irritating the lining of the throat and bronchi, inducing the production of excess mucous, sufferers frequently have the need to clear their throats and aspiration deeper into the lungs can result in chronic cough as the lungs attempt to expel the foreign matter.

In the lungs, it can cause asthma like symptoms. It can even build up resulting in pneumonia, bronchiectasis or idiopathic pulmonary fibrosis.

Causing irritation to the voice box, it can result in hoarseness and sore throat.

Attempting to prevent extra-oesophageal reflux, the cricopharyngeus may tighten or spasm producing a feeling of a lump in the throat known as Globus.

At night, in attempting to prevent reflux, the cricopharyngeus may be responsible for restricting breathing causing obstructive sleep apnoea.

Entering the mouth, reflux produces bad taste and bad breath. It can also cause dental erosion resulting in tooth decay or sharp edges to the teeth.

From the back of the throat, refluxate can travel via the eustachian tube to the ears where it may stimulate excessive wax production. This is more common in the right ear as lying on the right side results in more reflux than lying on the left. It can also result in tinnitus and peripheral vertigo (dizziness) and "glue ear" (otitis media).

Rising into the nasal chambers, excess mucous produced here can cause post nasal drip producing cough and result in the sufferer sniffing frequently to constrain it. This may also give rise to a poor sense of smell (hyposmia), a distortion of smell (parosmia) or even fool the senses to imagine smells that aren't there (phantosmia).

From the nasal passages, it can pass to the eyes via the tear ducts resulting in dry eye syndrome.

A 2014 poll of 100 reflux sufferers [r-i] revealed 70% reported experiencing hoarseness, 64% constant throat clearing, 58% post nasal drip, 58% chronic cough, 53% sinusitis, 53% bad taste in mouth, 50% globus (lump in throat), 42% asthma-like symptoms (shortness of breath), 41% tooth decay or sharp edges to teeth, 35% catarrhal symptoms (blocked nose), 35% Loss of voice, 35% dry or gritty eyes, 30% nocturnal ear waxing.

In other responses, the following symptoms were also highly indicated: bad breath, tinnitus, hyposmia (poor sense of smell), sore throat.

Following the findings of the 2014 poll, three fresh but interrelated surveys involving over 200 participants in 2017 [r-ii] rationalised the symptoms and explored the efficacy of PPIs and Anti-Reflux surgery on the management thereof.

Survey 1 targetting refluxers who didn't use daily pre-emptive medication but who may use occasional on-demand antacids as and when required garnered 51 responses.

Throat symptoms were most commonly identified with 63% reporting hoarseness, sore throat, loss of voice or throat clearing as a symptom. 45% reported globus, 43% post nasal drip, sinusitis or catarrh, 33% bad breath or taste in mouth, 31% dry or gritty eyes, 31% ear problems: waxing, glue ear, tinnitus or dizziness, 27% chest complaints, cough or asthma like symptoms and 22% dental problems.

Symptoms	Not taking regular medication	Taking regular medication
THROAT: Hoarseness, sore throat, loss of voice, throat clearing	63%	66%
CHEST: Chronic cough or asthma like symptoms	27%	46%
NOSE: Post nasal drip, Poor sense of smell, sinusitis, catarrhal symptoms	43%	49%
THROAT: Globus, feeling of lump in throat.	45%	50%
MOUTH: Tooth erosion	22%	26%
MOUTH: Bad breath or bad taste in mouth	33%	44%
EYES: Dry or gritty eyes	31%	42%
EARS: Waxing, Glue Ear, Tinnitus or dizziness	31%	48%

Survey 2 was completed by 100 refluxers using daily medication of H2 blockers or Proton Pump Inhibitors.

As with survey 1, the most prevalent reported symptom was concerned with the throat: hoarseness, sore throat, loss of voice and throat clearing reported by 66% of relfuxers with 50% reporting globus, 49% nasal problems, 48% ear problems, 46% cough, 44% oral, 42% eyes and 26% dental problems.

It is assumed those with the most prolific symptoms are the predominant users of acid suppressants (rather than PPIs actually result in higher incidence of EOR symptoms) and dosage levels seemed to make no difference.

Survey 3 targetted recipients of anti-reflux intervention. 52 responses were amassed during the collection period.
Pre intervention, 73% reported the throat issues and 58% globus with 50% reporting cough, 50% oral, 44% nasal, 35% aural, 33% eyes and 33% dental problems.

All but 2 repondees had received Nissen fundoplication, one had had Linx successfully and one had had Stretta unsuccessfully.

Post intervention, reported throat issues had been reduced to 35% oral problems 29%, globus 25%, cough 19% nasal problems 19%, eye problems 17%, ear problems 13% and dental erosion 10%.

A cumulative score of prevalence of symptoms reduced from 47% to 20% as a result of anti-reflux intervention.

Symptoms	Before intervention	After intervention
THROAT: Hoarseness, sore throat, loss of voice, throat clearing	73%	35%
CHEST: Chronic cough or asthma like symptoms	50%	19%
NOSE: Post nasal drip, Poor sense of smell, sinusitis, catarrhal symptoms	44%	19%
THROAT: Globus, feeling of lump in throat.	58%	25%
MOUTH: Tooth erosion	33%	10%
MOUTH: Bad breath or bad taste in mouth	50%	29%
EYES: Dry or gritty eyes	33%	17%
EARS: Waxing, Glue Ear, Tinnitus or dizziness	35%	13%

Conclusions

In the management of symptoms of extra-oesophageal reflux, acid suppressant medication did not appear to be effective whereas reflux reduction surgery was.

For those exhibiting symptoms of extra-oesophageal reflux, reflux reduction should be considered in preference to acid reduction.

A paper published in World Journal of Gastroenterology in May 2017 "Nissen fundoplication vs proton pump inhibitors for laryngopharyngeal reflux" [r-iii] using reviews of 53 patients, also concluded: "Laparoscopic Nissen Fundoplication achieves better improvement than PPIs for LPR."

To prevent reflux naturally

Think of the stomach as a balloon full of liquid. The Lower Oesophageal Sphincter should hold the neck tight shut. However, for some people it doesn't work as well as it should and the neck of the balloon isn't held as tightly as it should be.

If the balloon is over-full, squashed, shaken or tipped, the contents can spill.

So, to reduce reflux, we must ensure we do not over-fill the stomach. Eating little and often is the best way.

Excess body fat will press on the stomach so it may be necessary to lose weight. Tight clothing should also be avoided.

Exercise after food should only consist of gentle upright activity (eg walking which will help the food to pass through the stomach) and not involve bending down.

It is important to keep upright whilst the food moves through the stomach. Leave at least 3 hours between your last meal and going to bed.

By raising the head of the bed by 6 to 8 inches, gravity will help keep any residual contents in place and reflux is harder if you lie on your left side.

Reflux reduction

There aren't any easy drugs to combat reflux. Most people have to rely on lifestyle changes described above. The anti-emetic drugs, Domperidone and Metoclopramide may help some sufferers, however, and some people find their PPIs reduce reflux symptoms to some extent.

When lifestyle changes don't work, surgery may be an option.

The gold standard is Laparoscopic Nissen Fundoplication.

There are now, however, new devices, and treatments available that may prove effective in the future.

Section 4 – Treatments for reflux

Fundoplication

Fundoplication surgery involves stitching (or plicating) the top of the stomach (or fundus) around the base of the oesophagus to enhance the lower oesophageal sphincter and reduce reflux. There are various techniques available.

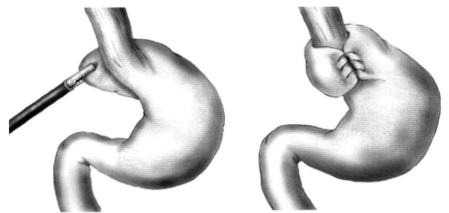

Diagram showing Nissen Fundoplication

Anterior 120º (or 90º etc)

To reduce the likelihood of inability to belch or vomit, or if the patient has motility problems, a partial wrap is favoured by some surgeons who will usually opt for a 120º wrap around the front (anterior) part of the oesophagus rather than a full 360º Nissen wrap.

Belsey

Dr Ronald Belsey's procedure was developed about the same time as the Nissen procedure and was the fundoplication of choice before the introduction of laparoscopic techniques. It is similar to a Nissen fundoplication though only performing a 270º wrap of the fundus around the oesophagus.
Since the surgery required access via the thorax rather than the abdomen, its popularity has been superceded by the Laparoscopic Nissen Fundoplication.

Collis

The Collis procedure isn't actually a fundoplication but is frequently accompanied by one. The procedure effectively produces an elongation of the oesophagus beneath the diaphragm into the stomach by sectioning the fundus. This often provides for a more effective Nissen or Belsey wrap which is frequently performed at the same time.

Dor

The Dor procedure is a 90° or 180° anterior wrap frequently employed in conjunction with a Heller's cardiomyotomy as a treatment for achalasia.

Heller's cardiomyotomy

Heller's cardiomyotomy isn't actually a fundoplication but is frequently accompanied by one.
The procedure may be used for patients suffering achalasia. By weakening or cutting the cardial muscles of the lower oesophageal sphincter, foods may pass more easily from the

oesophagus into the stomach. However, the opportunity for reflux may then be presented. To reduce that, a Dor partial fundoplication, or the similar Hill fundoplication, may be performed at the same time.

A paper published in the Annals of Surgery in 2006, stated: "Laparoscopic Heller myotomy allows the resolution of the dysphagia with minimal invasion, becoming the treatment of choice among surgeons and even gastroenterologists. The addition of an antireflux procedure to the esophageal myotomy is one of the major aspects of discussion between proponents of the anterior 90° (Dor) and the posterior 270° (Toupet) wrap, while there are some arguments against the routine use of an antireflux procedure." [f-i]

Nissen

With Hitler's rise to power, Rudolph Nissen, a Jewish doctor, fled his native Germany and, a few years later, Turkey, to America before returning after the war to Switzerland where he developed the gastric fundoplication procedure that now bears his name in 1954, having used similar techniques since 1937. Albert Einstein was one of his patients on whom he performed an operation to cure an aortic aneurysm - a later recurrence of which was to eventually kill him.

Nissen fundoplication has been used over the years on thousands of babies worldwide born with conditions that cause reflux disorders with lifetime results proving efficacy of the treatment.

Initially, inability to burp, belch or vomit was frequently encountered as a side effect but techniques have constantly been revised and developed which have minimised occurrence of these disturbing symptoms.

A Czech study published in 2013 [f-ii] stated ,"Anti-reflux operations are the only procedures which offer the possibility of treating the cause by restoring the anatomic barrier responsible for guarding against irritating effects of gastroduodenal content on the distal esophagus. Total (i.e. 360°) laparoscopic Nissen fundoplication (LNF) is considered the most effective amongst these procedures. Still, controversies related to the indications for anti-reflux surgery are frequently encountered. ...   Laparoscopic Nissen fundoplication, as a result of high effectiveness, represents the method of choice in the treatment of BE in the case of patients who were qualified for surgery."

In the 1990's laparoscopic (keyhole) surgery for fundoplication was introduced. Laparoscopic Nissen Fundoplication (LNF) is now considered the gold standard treatment for reflux against which all other techniques are evaluated.

A study published in Surgical Endoscopy in 2014 reviewed the durability of Laparoscopic Fundoplication over 20 years [f-iii] and concluded, "Long-term results from the early experience with LF are excellent with 94 % of patients reporting only occasional or fewer reflux symptoms at 20-year follow-up. However, 18 % required surgical revision surgery to maintain their results. There is a relatively high rate of daily dysphagia but 90 % of patients are happy to have had LF."

Rossetti

Dr. Mario Rossetti, a pupil of Rudolph Nissen, introduced a modification of the surgery in 1972, known as Nissen-Rossetti fundoplication, which utilises only the anterior wall of the fundus. Use of this modification is widespread.

A 2006 review of the procedure states, "When compared with other antireflux procedures, total fundoplication is the most effective barrier against reflux. Nissen-Rossetti, in particular, achieves this goal without the need to resection the short gastric vessels." [f-iv]

Toupet

Unlike other partial wraps, that developed by André Toupet in 1963 is a 270° posterior wrap of the fundus around the back of the oesophagus designed to reduce dysphagia and the occurrence of a hiatus hernia.

A paper published in International Surgery in 2003, stated, "for patients in whom esophageal peristalsis is documented to be weak preoperatively, use of a partial wrap, or Toupet procedure, has often been used as an alternative to lessen the potential for postoperative dysphagia" and concluded, "We recommend its selective use in patients with preoperative esophageal hypomotility who are undergoing laparoscopic antireflux surgery." [f-v]

Footnotes

Although the main variations of fundoplication surgery have been included above, there are and have been other modifications to the Nissen fundoplication not described here, including those performed by Drs Phillip Donahue, Pearson and Henderson, Orringer and Sloan, Thomas Bombeck, Lucian Hill and Thomas DeMeester.

The Medscape overview of fundoplication (2014) says, "When comparing the efficacy of antireflux surgery with medical treatment, there has been considerable debate. A systematic review concluded similar efficacy between these 2 treatment options. Some recent literature suggests that long-term outcomes from antireflux surgery may be superior to medical treatment. The latest guidelines from the American College of Gastroenterology indicate, "surgical therapy is as effective as medical therapy for carefully selected patients with chronic GERD when performed by an experienced surgeon" (strong recommendation; high level of evidence). In appropriately selected patients, laparoscopic reflux surgery may be more cost effective than lifelong medical treatment." [f-vi]

See Appendix 1 for the NICE Options Grid to aid patient discussion regarding fundoplication vs medication.

LINX

The LINX band is a bracelet of magnetic titanium beads inserted around the Oesophagus to augment the Lower Oesophageal Sphincter. These images, from the manufacturer's (Torax medical) website, show how it works.

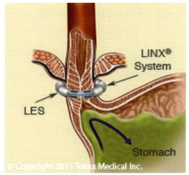 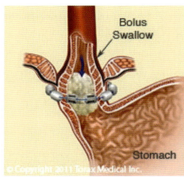 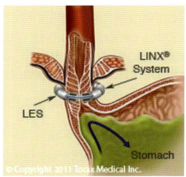

1. The LINX® system helps the LOS resist opening to gastric pressures. 2. It expands to allow for normal swallowing. 3. Magnetic attraction closes the LOS immediately after swallowing.

But while it looks like the best alternative to Nissen fundoplication presently, there are also some concerns.

It has been heavily promoted on the possible adverse effects of Nissen fundoplication and it has gained free media attention in the United States whenever another clinic offers this new device. But whereas they have been quick to point to possible shortcomings of Nissen fundoplication, the manufacturers do not so readily publicise the possible adverse effects of the device leading one journal to produce an article: "Heartburn Hell on the NBC Today Show: omitting things consumers might want to know about a $14K device" in response to one such publicity feature. [r-ii]

Long term results aren't available yet.

A report in the Journal of American College of Surgeons highlighted on the Torax website, "One Hundred Consecutive Patients Treated with Magnetic Sphincter Augmentation for Gastroesophageal Reflux Disease: 6 Years of Clinical Experience from a Single Center" [r-iii] examined results of patients having had the implant an average of 3 years.

It concluded "Magnetic sphincter augmentation for GERD in clinical practice provides safe and long-term reduction of esophageal acid exposure, substantial symptom improvement, and elimination of daily PPI use." and "Freedom from daily dependence on PPIs was achieved in 85% of patients."

The report also included the reasons patients gave for choosing the device instead of Nissen fundoplication saying they believed the alternative was "effective only in the short-term, too invasive, resulted in dysphagia, inability to belch/vomit and was not reversible".

The approval of the FDA in America, coupled with the positive news items, has meant a surge in demand for the device but patients have found a reluctance on the part of insurance companies to pay for it. Most commercial insurers still see the LINX as too new to cover. Spokespeople with Aetna and Blue Cross and Blue Shield of Minnesota said they consider the device "investigational," needing further study. [r-iv]

A report from the University of Southern California [r-v], revealed that 63% of LINX recipients experienced difficulty swallowing following implantation. The problem being the bolus of food travelling down the oesphagus needs to be dense enough and propelled strongly enough by the patient's peristalsis to push the magnets apart.

NICE guidelines [r-vi] permit the use of LINX "with special arrangements for clinical governance, consent and audit or research" because "the evidence on the safety and efficacy of laparoscopic insertion of a magnetic bead band for gastro-oesophageal reflux disease (GORD) is limited in quantity". The cost to NHS is double that of a Laparoscopic Nissen Fundoplication so the availability of LINX on the NHS is currently limited, but it's available privately. The price for private treatment is in the region of £8,000-£9,000.

A study published in Annals of Surgery May 2016, followed 164 LINX recipients over 48 months. [r-ix] of whom 11 had the device explanted: 2 having experienced fill thickness erosion of the device through the oesophageal wall.

Another paper published in June 2017 [r-x] reported another 2 cases of migration of the device through the oesophageal wall.

A paper published in May 2017 found LINX more effective than PPIs for treating regurgitation in GERD. [r-xi]

Stretta

The Stretta procedure uses radio frequency energy bursts to tighten the lower oesophageal sphincter to help it function correctly.

The manufacturers state, *"We do not position Stretta as competitive treatment with surgery – but instead a less invasive bridge that allows some patients for whom medications are not completely effective to avoid surgery and its potential complications, or if someone has had surgery allows them an option other than additional surgery."*

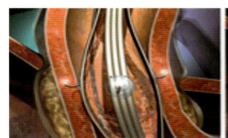 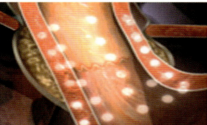 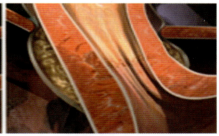

From the manufacturer's (Mederi Therapeutics) own website, www.stretta-therapy.com:

> When patients suffer from chronic gastroesophageal reflux disease (GERD) that is not well controlled with medications, or where long-term medications are not a viable option, Stretta offers an alternative other than surgery and implants. Stretta is a unique and minimally invasive outpatient procedure that takes about an hour, with patients returning to normal activities within a few days.
> - Studies show that Stretta resolves reflux symptoms and improves quality of life
> - Stretta reduces or eliminates medications and reduces acid exposure
> - A minimally invasive option that is less aggressive than invasive surgery and implants
> - More than 33 clinical studies all conclude Stretta is "safe and effective"
> - Stretta results are long-lasting, proven effective from 4-10 years
> - Treats the underlying cause of GERD not just the symptoms
> Stretta is an important part of the continuum of care for patients with chronic GERD and is the ideal "middle therapy" fitting between medicine and surgery, yet not preventing a patient from moving on to more invasive options in the future if necessary.

A 10 year follow-up report of patients who had received Stretta therapy published in Surgical Endoscopy February 2014 [r-xii] showed "72 % of patients normalizing GERD symptom scores, 41 % of patients able to remain off regular medication for GERD, 64 % of patients able to reduce medication use by 50 % or greater, and more than 60 % sustained improvement in satisfaction."

In the USA, SAGES (Society of American Gastrointestinal and Endoscopic Surgeons) guidelines issued June 2013 [r-xiii] recommended "Stretta is considered appropriate therapy for patients being treated for GERD who are 18 years of age or older, who have had symptoms of heartburn, regurgitation, or both for 6 months or more, who have been partially or completely responsive to anti-secretory pharmacologic therapy, and who have declined laparoscopic fundoplication."

Stretta may be recommended as an appropriate therapeutic option for patients with GERD who meet current indications and patient selection criteria and choose endoluminal therapy over laparoscopic fundoplication. Those criteria include:

Adult patients (age >=18) with symptoms of heartburn, regurgitation, or both for >= 6 months who have been partially or completely responsive to antisecretory pharmacologic therapy.

The procedure has not been studied and should not be applied in treating patients with severe esophagitis, hiatus hernias > 2 cm, long segment Barrett esophagus, dysphagia, or those with a history of autoimmune disease, collagen vascular disease, and/or coagulation disorders. Further studies are needed to evaluate the role of Stretta in children if it is to be considered a therapeutic option.

In UK, NICE have yet to rule on it's use. *"NICE has been notified about the above procedure and are currently undertaking preliminary investigations, with the aim of assessing whether this procedure falls within the remit of the Interventional Procedures Programme."*

N.B. This procedure is not to be confused with Radio Frequency Ablation.

Transoral Incisionless Fundoplication

60 years of fundoplication have proved its efficacy in reducing reflux. For the last 20 years the operation has been performed laparoscopically offering minimal invasive surgery.

There have been many attempts to develop a method of performing fundoplication via the oesophagus itself - endoluminal gastroplication.

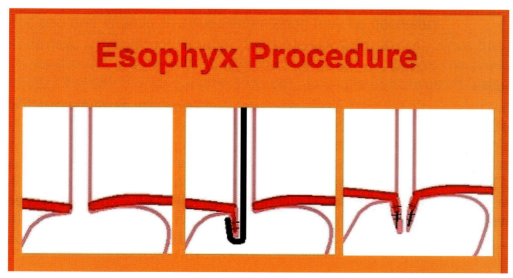

The Esophyx® Transoral Incisionless Fundoplication device by Endogastric Solutions "enables the creation of a 2-3 cm, 270° esophogastric fundoplication by using proprietary tissue manipulating elements and 12 or more full-thickness polypropylene fasteners. The device is used in conjunction with a flexible video endoscope, which provides visualization throughout the TIF® procedure."

An article in World Journal of Surgery in 2008, "Anti-reflux Transoral Incisionless Fundoplication using EsophyX: 12-month results of a Prospective Multicenter study," written by surgeons employed by Endogastric solutions, concluded, "12-month results showed that EsophyX-TIF was safe and effective in improving quality of life and for reducing symptoms." [r-xiv]
This helped the device get FDA approval for use in the US.

However, the paper also stated, "Global assessment revealed that 56% of patients were "cured" of their GERD based on the clinically significant reduction of their heartburn and complete cessation off PPIs."

The fastener technique was being revised at this stage to produce Esophyx®2 with this optimistic message: "The tailored fastener placement technique (TIF2.0) is expected to further improve on these results and support the use of EsophyX-TIF for the treatment of GERD."

In 2009, another Endogastric solutions sponsored study published in Surgical Endoscopy [r-xv] reporting "Two-year results of a feasibility study on antireflux transoral incisionless fundoplication using Esophyx" concluded: "The results at 2 years supported the long-term safety and durability of TIF and its sustained effect on the elimination of heartburn, esophagitis, ≤2 cm hiatal hernia, and daily dependence on PPIs" with "a ≥50% improvement in GERD-HRQL scores compared with those at baseline on PPIs was sustained by 64% of patients."

A 2011 paper, "Clinical and pH-metric outcomes of transoral esophagogastric fundoplication for the treatment of gastroesophageal reflux disease," [r-xvi] funded by Endogastric solutions, concluded: "using the EsophyX device significantly improved symptomatic and objective outcomes in over 70% of patients at median 6-month follow-up."

A review by MedGadget in 2013, "EsophyX for Transoral Incisionless Fundoplication (TIF) Proves Itself in Trial" [r-xvii] reported, "Twenty-four months after the EsophyX2® device was used in TIF procedures, more than two-thirds of patients completely eliminated the need for daily proton pump inhibitor (PPIs) therapy. Symptom control achieved at six months remained stable over time indicating durability of TIF procedure."

A 2014 report published in the American Journal of Gastroenterology and reported in Medscape, "TIF Underperforming as Long-Term GERD Treatment" [r-xviii], concluded: "Although TIF resulted in an improved GERD-related quality of life and produced a short-term improvement of the antireflux barrier in a selected group of GERD patients, no long-term objective reflux control was achieved." Further, one of the doctors commentating on the findings stated, "Numerous uncontrolled trials have demonstrated rapid deterioration of TIF results. Since the TIF procedure does not allow mobilization of the gastric fundus, tension on the wrap causes the TIF fasteners to pull apart. The TIF procedure has no proven long-term benefit."

MUSE™ Medigus Ultrasonic Surgical Endostapler

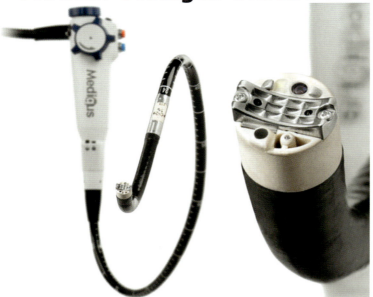

Similar in concept to the Esophyx TIF system described above, the Israeli developed MUSE stapler is newer and still undergoing initial trials with first MUSE procedures performed in Turkey [r-xix] and Italy [r-xx].

It uses a special endoscope equipped with a stapler, video camera, light source, ultrasound, water spray and suction.

The tip of the stapler, guided by the video system, is bent round the fundus section at the gastro-oesophageal junction until too close to see clearly when the ultrasound takes over to ensure the staple is positioned through the correct tissue thickness.

A paper, "Endoscopic anterior fundoplication with the Medigus Ultrasonic Surgical Endostapler (MUSE™) for gastroesophageal reflux disease: 6-month results from a multi-center prospective trial" funded by Medigus, published in Surgical Endoscopy in 2014 [r-xxi], concluded: "The initial 6-month data reported in this study demonstrate safety and efficacy of this endoscopic plication device. Early experience with the device necessitated procedure and device changes to improve safety, with improved results in the later portion of the study."

As a result of this study, the system was FDA cleared and CE marked for endoscopic placement of surgical staples in the soft tissue of the esophagus and stomach.
NICE guidance on Endoluminal Gastroplication for Gastro-Oesophageal Reflux Disease [r-xxii] says, "The evidence on endoluminal gastroplication for gastro-oesophageal reflux disease (GORD) raises no major safety concerns. Evidence from a number of randomised controlled trials (RCTs) shows a degree of efficacy in terms of reduced medication requirement in the short term, but changes in other efficacy outcomes are inconsistent and there is no good evidence of sustained improvement in oesophageal pH measurements. Therefore, this procedure should only be used with special arrangements for clinical governance, consent and audit or research."

EndoCinch™

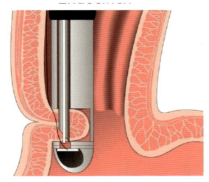

The earliest form of endoluminal gastroplication was the EndoCinch which quickly gained FDA approval in USA.

It pulled some of the wall of the esophagus into a chamber at the end of a special endoscope where it was plicated (stitched) to form pleats.

Early reports were favourable. In 2003, the British Medical Journal, Gut reported: "The Endocinch procedure is an effective and safe outpatient procedure that offers GORD patients significant improvement in symptomatology, QOL, and reduced requirements for PPIs over at least a one year period." [r-xxiii]

However, a couple of years later, the same journal reported a different story:

" Endoscopic gastroplication (EndoCinch) is a safe and minimally invasive endoscopic treatment for GORD with reasonable short term results. In contrast, long term outcome is disappointing, probably due to suture loss in the majority of patients. Therefore, technical improvements to ensure suture durability are mandatory before endoscopic suturing can evolve as a therapeutic option for GORD treatment." [r-xxiv]

In 2007, another Gut article reported: "the retention of stitches seems to be a major problem reported with this technique" referenced in a Healthline item [r-xxv] which also reported a German study of 2005 that recommended that, "even though it's considered safe and easy to perform, EndoCinch endoluminal gastroplication shouldn't be used as a treatment for gastroesophageal reflux disease 'until further technical refinements allow sutures to be maintained in the long term.'"

The manufacturers Bard, have since stopped producing the device.

Endogastric Solutions (who now market the Esophyx® TIF device described above), developed Stomaphyx® using a similar technique to suture the connection between the stomach pouch and small intestines resulting in slower emptying of the stomach and earlier satiety and more weight loss also shrinking the stomach pouch and making it small, similar to the outcome of the original gastric bypass surgery." However, like EndoCinch, long term outcomes showed the procedure wasn't durable. [r-xxvi]

NICE guidlines on Endoluminal gastroplication for gastro-oesophageal reflux disease [r-xxvii] state, "The evidence on endoluminal gastroplication for gastro-oesophageal reflux disease (GORD) raises no major safety concerns. Evidence from a number of randomised controlled trials (RCTs) shows a degree of efficacy in terms of reduced medication requirement in the short term, but changes in other efficacy outcomes are inconsistent and there is no good evidence of sustained improvement in oesophageal pH measurements. Therefore, this procedure should only be used with special arrangements for clinical governance, consent and audit or research."

Endostim

Sometimes referred to as "The Pacemaker for the Lower Oesophageal Sphincter", Endostim is a new treatment which had its first clinical trial in 2010.

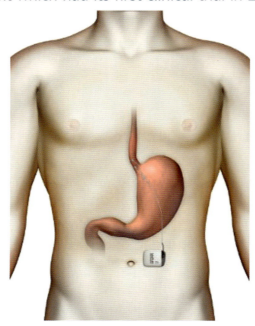

An electrical stimulator is placed in the abdomen with leads to the muscles of the lower oesophageal sphincter.

It uses low energy electrical impulses to strengthen a weak or improperly functioning lower oesophageal sphincter muscle to restore the natural anti-reflux barrier between the stomach and oesophagus without interfering with normal oesophageal function such as swallowing.

In January 2012, a report published in Neuorgastroenterology and Motility following initial experimentation [r-xxviii], concluded: "Short-term stimulation of the LES in patients with GERD significantly increases resting LESP without affecting esophageal peristalsis or LES relaxation. Electrical stimulation of the LES may offer a novel therapy for patients with GERD."

A paper published in Surgical Endoscopy in October 2012 [r-xxix] reported on a pilot trial: "Electrical stimulation of the lower esophageal sphincter (LES) improves LES pressure without interfering with LES relaxation. The aim of this open-label pilot trial was to evaluate the safety and efficacy of long-term LES stimulation using a permanently implanted LES stimulator in patients with gastroesophageal reflux disease (GERD)."

A report was published on PR Newswire in February 2013 of the first patient being treated in Germany. [r-xxx]

A paper published in Endoscopy in 2013 [r-xxxi] concluded: "During the long term follow-up of 12 months, LES–EST was safe and effective for the treatment of GERD. There was a significant and sustained improvement in GERD symptoms, reduction in esophageal acid exposure with elimination of daily PPI usage, and no stimulation-related adverse effects."

"Two-year results of intermittent electrical stimulation of the lower esophageal sphincter treatment of gastroesophageal reflux disease" were published in Surgery in March 2015 [r-xxxii] concluding, "LES-EST is safe and effective for treating patients with GERD over a period of 2 years. LES-EST resulted in a significant and sustained improvement in GERD symptoms, and esophageal acid exposure and eliminated PPI use in majority of patients (16 of 21). Further, LES-EST was not associated with any gastrointestinal side effects or adverse events."

In March 2015, PR Newswire reported Endostim had released a "second generation" stimulator that was smaller in size with "improved MRI conditional compatibility for head and extremity imaging procedures, adding support for 3T MRI machines in addition to the 1.5T MRI machines." [r-xxxiii]

NICE has been notified about this procedure and is developing guidance on it. [r-xxxiv]

Enteryx

The idea behind Enteryx is simple. Inject a bulking agent into the walls of the oesophagus near the junction with the stomach to enhance the lower oesophageal sphincter.

Patient trials were commenced in 2002 with great hopes. It was approved by FDA in America in April 2003.

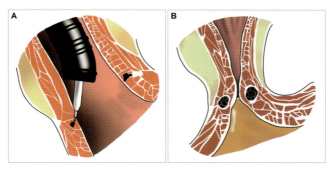

In September 2003 a research paper published in the American Journal of Gastroenterology [r-xxxv] concluded: "Enteryx implantation allows most patients to discontinue PPI therapy, improves their symptoms, and reduces esophageal acid exposure. The effects of implantation are long-lasting, and morbidity is transient and minimal. The procedure requires basic endoscopic skills and seems to provide a useful option in the effective clinical management of GERD."

A paper published in Gastrointestinal Endoscopy in 2005 [r-xxxvi] stated: "In conclusion, this report encompasses a large cohort of patients with PPI-dependent GERD treated with Enteryx implantation into the distal esophagus. The findings indicate that Enteryx is a safe, effective, and durable endoluminal therapy for the majority of treated patients." However, the same publication reported a case study where complications had occurred. [r-xxxvii]

In October 2005, the FDA issued a Preliminary Public Health Notification [r-xxxviii] and the manufacturers recalled the device.

The Journal of Radiology Case Reports in 2014 published an account whereby the bulking agent had been injected into the visceral artery. [r-xxxix]

It noted: "Endoscopic injection of Enteryx into the lower esophageal sphincter carries the risk of inadvertent intravascular injection and migration of the polymer into visceral arteries. Although the product has been withdrawn from the market, similar products may be developed in the future and operators need to be aware of the potential complications of such injection and the risks of intravascular embolization. A test in which contrast is injected before the polymer mixture can help ascertain the location of injection and improve the safety of the procedure."

Gatekeeper

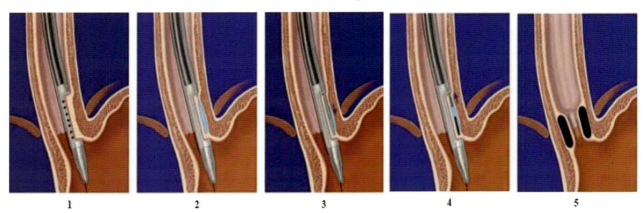

The Gatekeeper procedure:

1. The oesophagus wall is aspirated. 2. Normal saline is injected into the sub-mucosal layer. 3. A pocket is created in the sub-mucosal layer. 4. The prosthesis is implanted in the pocket. 5. View after completion of the operation.

Instead of injecting a polymer like Enteryx, Gatekeeper placed a hydrogel rod just under the surface of the oesophagus.

However problems occurred with the prosthesis remaining in situ. The device never received approval from NICE whose guidance on the procedure in 2007 [r-xl] stated *"There is limited evidence of short-term efficacy on endoscopic augmentation of the lower oesophageal sphincter using hydrogel implants for the treatment of gastro-oesophageal reflux disease (GORD). This evidence also raises concerns about the procedure's safety. Therefore, this procedure should not be used without special arrangements for consent and for audit"* and it is no longer available.

Angelchik

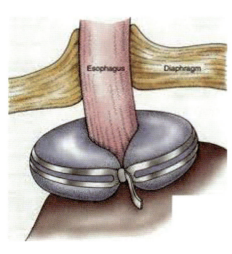

In 1973 a new device was used for the first time to reduce GERD (although not in general use until 1979). Effectively a rubber band around the oeosphagus, Angelchik would supplement the lower oesophageal sphincter and prevent reflux misery.

"It consisted of a C-shaped ring of silicon fitted around the gastroesophageal junction. The ring was secured in place by means a fitted Dacron tape. It was well favored at the time compared to other antireflux surgeries because of the simple and standardized technique of insertion of the device. Over 25,000 devices were inserted worldwide." [r-xli]

"The main advantage was the ease of insertion with low morbidity and short hospital stay. Its efficacy by 24-hour pH-metry and/or manometry was confirmed in several studies that suggested that the Angelchik ring provides early postoperative control." [r-xlii]

By 1984, there were signs all may not be as good as was originally thought:

"Various complications have been reported recently for the Angelchik antireflux prosthesis, a silicone-gel prosthesis used in the treatment of gastroesophageal reflux and associated hiatal hernia. We have studied the cases of 11 patients with complications of this prosthesis and have reviewed the literature for others. Complications included 8 erosions of the device into the gastrointestinal tract, 1 migration, 1 improper placement, and 1 case of pain believed to be a sequela of surgical trauma. These complications represent those typical to reflux surgery and some unique to the Angelchik prosthesis (migration and erosion). Their exact frequency is unknown, with the manufacturer estimating migration at 0.81% and erosion at 0.15%. Available data indicate that complications may occur up to several years after implantation, and physicians may not recognize the problems with the prosthesis if they are unaware of the complications." [r-xliii]

"Enthusiasm for the device hugely subsided when long-term results became available. Up to 70% of patients developed moderate to severe dysphagia. In addition, other complications were frequently reported including migration of the device (due to Dacron tape failure) and erosion into surrounding structures.

"By 1990, use of the Angelchik device was almost entirely abandoned and open Nissen's fundoplication became the accepted technique to treat GERD. Nowadays the laparoscopic version of this procedure is common place." [r-xli]

New non-surgical treatments for extra-oesophageal reflux: Reza Band

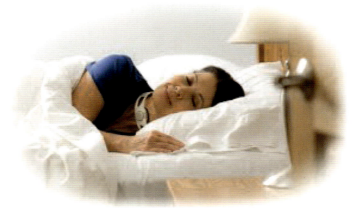

Reza Band from Somna Therapeutics is a device worn around the neck at night to provide sufficient pressure on the cricopharyngeus muscle to prevent nocturnal extra-oesophageal reflux.

The results of a limited clinical trial published in Gastroenterology in 2012 [r-xliv], revealed, "All patients tolerated the device well and completed the study. There were no complications or complaints for the use of the device."

A questionnaire is provided for prospective users. (Compare the list of symptoms described in the chapter on Extra-Oesophageal Reflux).

Are you Affected by these problems? If so, rate them from 0 (No problem) to 5 (Severe problem).

> Hoarseness or a problem with your voice
> Clearing your throat
> Excess throat mucous or postnasal drip
> Difficulty swallowing food, liquids, or pills
> Coughing after eating or after lying down
> Breathing difficulties
> Troublesome or annoying cough
> Sensations of something sticking in your throat or a lump in your throat
> Heartburn, chest pain, indigestion, or stomach acid coming up

Total your score.

A total score of more than 13 is considered a positive diagnosis of acid reflux in the throat and lungs.

MedClineTM

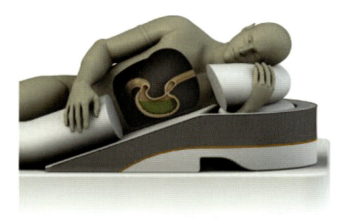

To reduce nocturnal reflux, patients are advised to raise their bed head or use a wedge pillow and to sleep on their left side.

MedCline is a device designed to make that easier to achieve.

A paper published by the Cleveland Clinic in 2014 [r-xlv] conlcuded, "In patients with nocturnal heartburn and regurgitation despite PPI use, the Medcline Sleep Positioning Device significantly reduced nocturnal symptoms, morning impact of nocturnal GERD, and concern about nocturnal GERD after two weeks of use."

A paper published in the American Journal of Gastroenterology in 2015 [r-xlvi], concluded, "The sleep positioning device maintains recumbent position effectively. Lying left-side down, it reduces recumbent esophageal acid exposure."

Section 5 – Food

Acid and Alkali foods
The acidity or alkalinity of what we consume actually has little or no bearing on the acid production of the stomach.
Stomach acid is produced by the parietal cells in the stomach in response to action of neurotransmitters histamine and acetylcholine. It is highly concentrated hydrochloric acid that can dissolve metal.
If you pour vinegar (an acid) on your hand, it will feel wet. Pour battery acid on your hand and it will cause damage. Pour vinegar on the damaged area and it will hurt; it's not the vinegar that's caused the problem but the concentrated acid.
Despite the many articles on "health" websites extolling the values of alkaline diets, they do nothing to reduce stomach acid.
Acidity is measured in terms of pH. pH7 is neutral: anything below is acid and anything above is alkaline.
Stomach acid "at rest" is usually pH4 but can reach pH1 when "active". (Vinegar is pH4.)
You can measure pH values using indicator papers but, whereas saliva or urine may be easily measured, stomach acid cannot.

Foods that may cause reflux
Some drugs (like caffeine and alcohol) may cause the muscles of the lower oesophageal sphincter to relax which could exacerbate reflux. However, for those experiencing frequent reflux, their sphincter is obviously malfunctioning anyway and the drugs' actions may make little difference.
Anything causing a build up of gas in the stomach may cause reflux.
This includes beans, brassicas (cabbage, cauliflower, etc), salad vegetables (cucumbers, radishes etc), fruits, grains, dairy products, breads and cereals etc.
Perhaps sounding counter-intuitve, sipping plain soda water can help by permitting a controlled burp to release the gas.

Know your triggers
Some acid refluxers may be affected by some foods. They are their trigger foods.
However, as everyone is different, not everyone is affected in the same way by the same foods. We don't know why some foods act as a trigger for some and not others. It could be to do with the foods we were weaned on, our environment or even the food choice of our mothers whilst we were still in the womb.
To determine your food triggers, you should keep a food diary writing down the components and times of meals and recording any possible consequences. Analysing your log after a week or two may identify common elements that caused your reflux.
These items are frequently found on people's trigger foods lists but they may not affect you. If unaffected, you don't need to avoid them:
Spicy Foods, Citrus fruits, tomatoes, dairy products, fatty foods, soda, coffee.

Some food myths

Coffee. Although the caffeine content may relax the sphincter, research has shown that for most acid refluxers, coffee need not be avoided.
There have been a number of studies looking at the effects of coffee.
A study of over 8000 patients in Japan in 2012 [fd-i] found "No association of coffee consumption with gastric ulcer, duodenal ulcer, reflux esophagitis, and non-erosive reflux disease."
And a study published by American Gastroenterological Association in May 2016 [fd-ii] found "Coffee or Tea, Hot or Cold, Are Not Associated With Risk of Barrett's Esophagus."

Alcohol. A search through the Barrett's Wessex accumulated archive of research links relevant to reflux, Barrett's etc, from all reputable journals over the last 5+ years [fd-iii], found 9 studies showing alcohol had no harmful effect on Barrett's Oesophagus:
"alcohol consumption is not a risk factor" (Gut 2005)
"No significant effects of alcohol consumption" (Digestive Diseases & Sciences 2013)
"Alcohol drinking is not associated with risk of neoplastic progression in Barrett's esophagus." (PLoS one 2014)
"we found no evidence that alcohol consumption increases the risk of Barrett's esophagus." (American Journal of Gastroenterology 2014)
"alcohol consumption ... [did] not seem to have any impact" (Gastroenterology Research & Practice 2014)
"Alcohol consumption ... [is] not associated with the condition." (Gastrointestinal Tumors 2016)
In fact 2 studies seemed to show it may actually have a beneficial effect.
"Significant inverse association was observed between alcohol consumption and BE," (Medicine Baltimore 2016)
"The limited data available on alcohol consumption supports a tentative inversion of alcohol consumption with BE risk in women" (Scientific Reports 2015)
(Alcohol was, however, considered to have a detrimental effect on the development of squamous cell cancer.)

Alkaline Water. Heavily promoted by those who hope to profit from its sale, only one study has shown any positive effects from alkaline water [fd-iv]. It was not replicated by peer review and not produced by a gastroenterologist but an ENT specialist who may be a beneficiary of companies selling the product.
These articles have debunked any claims alkaline water may provide:
Alkaline Water Hoax [fd-v]
Alkaline Water Helps neutralize Heartburn Symptoms? Doctors Debunk Claims [fd-vi]
The Doctor is in: Water, water everywhere - which drop should we drink? [fd-vii]

How we eat is important

Our modern lifestyle is much to blame for an increase in acid reflux and its associated problems.

We are prone to eat too much and too quickly and probably the wrong foods, too. (For instance fatty or processed meats need longer to break down in the stomach so should not be eaten in a rush, "on the go".)

When we eat, we need to eat small portions to avoid over-filling the stomach. We should eat slowly to permit each food bolus to enter the stomach and start being processed before the next is sent on its way.

Chewing each mouthful well will stimulate secretion of saliva and mucous to protect and lubricate the oesophagus to facilitate peristalsis to the stomach.

Keeping upright whilst eating is important for gravity to help.

A 1999 study on The role of diet and lifestyle measures in the pathogenesis and treatment of gastroesophageal reflux disease [fd-viii] stated, "A general consensus on the control of GERD through alterations in diet and lifestyle factors could hardly be based on the results of clinical or outcome studies."

This was further supported by a 2017 study Diet and GERD: Role in Pathogenesis and Management [fd-ix] stating, "Although anecdotal evidence has suggested associations with certain foods (fats, nonvegetarian, fried foods, and beverages) with reflux symptoms, objective evidence based data in this field remain unclear. Recent evidence points to the increasing importance of lifestyle in disease development as well."

And this item [fd-x] said, "It's Not Food Causing Your Heartburn—Here Are The 5 Real Culprits"

Exercise after food

After eating, the stomach should be allowed to empty before any activity which would result in it being squeezed, tilted or shaken.

It is probably best to abstain from activities like sit-ups, heavy lifting, bending down, running, swimming etc for an hour after eating.

However, gentle upright exercise is encouraged like walking which will help the food move from the stomach into the duodenum quicker.

Section 6 – Combinations and Complications

Oesophagitis

The mucosa lining the oesophagus produces mucous to aid movement of food to the stomach and to provide some protection to the surface layer (epithelium) of the oesophagus. However, acid refluxing can wash away some of the mucosal protection and come into contact with the lining itself. This is highly concentrated hydrochloric acid; strong enough to be able to dissolve metal, if you were to spill some on your hand it was cause significant scarring - which it can also do to the oesophagus.
We may feel the acid burning as heartburn (though 30% with persistent acid reflux report never having felt it).

Inflammation and scarring caused by the acid is called oesophagitis. Sometimes an endoscopist will classify the degree of oesophagitis observed using one of the following scales:

The Savary-Miller grading system is commonly used:

Grade 1: single or multiple erosions on a single fold. Erosions may ooze fluids or just show redness.
Grade 2: multiple erosions affecting multiple folds. Erosions may be joined together.
Grade 3: multiple circumferential erosions.
Grade 4: ulceration, narrowing or oesophageal shortening.
Grade 5: Barrett's epithelium. Columnar metaplasia in the form of circular or non-circular (islands or tongues) and extensions.

The more recent and more objective Los Angeles grades A to D classification is also used.

Grade A: one or more mucosal breaks no longer than 5 mm, none of which extends between the tops of the mucosal folds.
Grade B: one or more mucosal breaks more than 5 mm long, none of which extends between the tops of two mucosal folds.
Grade C: mucosal breaks that extend between the tops of two or more mucosal folds, but which involve <75% of the mucosal circumference
Grade D: mucosal breaks which involve ≥75% of the mucosal circumference

Barrett's Oeosphagus

Combinations of Acid. Bile and Reflux may have various complications and associated disorders which are discussed within this chapter, including Barrett's Oesophagus which can progress to cancer.

Acid Reflux → Oesophagitis → **Barrett's Oesophagus** → Oesophageal cancer

Acid refluxing into the oesophagus may wash aside the mucous lining and attack the squamous cells beneath - in the same way as pouring acid on your hand would burn and scar. This may be felt as heartburn and continued erosion can result in **oesophagitis**.

If bile refluxes onto the inflamed area, it could start to digest the exposed lining in the same way as it would break down ingested animal products. As a protection, the squamous cells can be replaced by columnar cells.

An analogy is to think of squamous cells as dominoes lying on a table. Columnar cells are like dominoes standing on end with a smaller surface exposed to attack. Meanwhile the nerves centred within the cells are further moved from the attack so these cells are effectively less sensitive and the misery of heartburn may diminish. These cells resemble those that line the stomach or intestines and may be described as gastric or intestinal metaplasia.

The Domino metaphor

Healthy Oesophagus lined with flat "squamous" cells

Barrett's Oesophagus lined with "columnar" cells

Dysplasia columnar cells mutate

(Cancer = an unco-ordinated pile)

(There is some discussion as to whether Barrett's cells are actually "metaplasia", which infers they are changed squamous cells or whether they are actually new cells produced from stem cells - as discussed in a July 2017 paper "Barrett's Stem Cells as a Unique and Targetable Entity" [c-i])

This is the condition known as **Barrett's Oesophagus** and it is a permanent change. Sometimes Barrett's appears to go away but if it's not seen, it may be hidden in the corrugations of the epithelium or a second mucosal layer may have grown over it. The burning sensations may reduce or disappear adding to the illusion that the Barrett's has gone but Barrett's itself is asymptomatic and the cells being less sensitive are protecting against the pain.

However, these cells are unregulated and in a small minority of cases can mutate. In our analogy, it's like some of the dominoes toppling. This is called Low Grade Dysplasia (LGD).

If a large mass of these dominoes topples into a disorganised heap, it's known as High Grade Dysplasia (HGD).

Further mutations may now occur which can cause a proliferation of mutated cells which is **Oesophageal Adenocarcinoma** - *that's cancer!*

The different stages of Barrett's Oesophagus are:

1. Non-Dysplastic Barrett's Oesophagus (NDBO/NDBE)
    2. Low Grade Dysplasia (LGD)
    3. High Grade Dysplasia (HGD)
    4. Neoplasia - initial stage of adenocarcinoma. (OAC/EAC)

The phrase "Indefinite for Dysplasia" is often used if there is uncertainty whether it's NDBO or LGD.

It must be stressed that the chances of progression of Barrett's Oesophagus to Oesophageal cancer are very low and *it is treatable.*

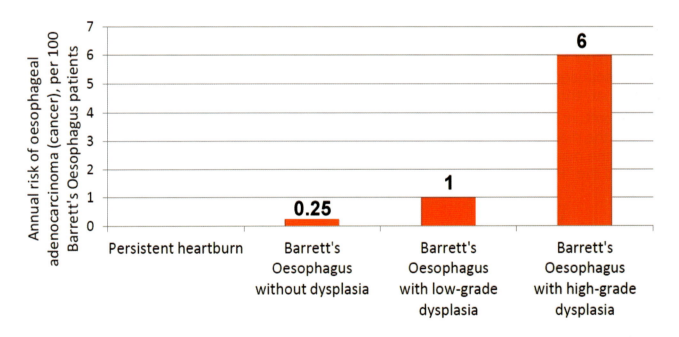

(Just under 8000 people die each year from Oesophageal Cancer out of 64 million in UK, making the chances one in 8000. If there are 3 million with non-dysplasic Barrett's*, their risk is one in 400.)

Britain tops the world for incidence of oesophageal cancer where it is the fifth greatest cancer killer of men, claiming the life of one person an hour on average in the UK. [c-ii]

If it is going to occur, the progression is usually slow initially but by the time cancerous cells develop, it's frequently too late to treat with life expectancy measured in weeks rather than years.

A paper published in 2014 [c-iii] suggests one in 20 have Barrett's. Applying that to the UK population implies there may be 3 million people with Barrett's though fewer than 150,000 know it. If the others can be identified, it may be possible to prevent this large number of deaths.

Prague classification.

The size and extent of an observed area of Barrett's may be described using the Prague criteria using the letters **c** for circumferential ring and **m** for maximum length of any tongues. Thus c2m3 would mean a ring of Barrett's 2 cm wide with protrusions to a maximum of 3 cm.

How Barrett's Oesophagus Forms – put simply

Your stomach is like this water balloon but instead of water, it holds very concentrated hydrochloric acid and instead of fingers holding the top closed, there are two sets of muscles at the base of the ribcage, together known as the Lower Oesophageal Sphincter (or LOS).

If you tip or squeeze the balloon when it's full, it will leak unless it is held tightly closed. With the stomach, that would mean concentrated acid leaking into the tube above, the oesophagus, which it may attack and is frequently experienced as heartburn or acid reflux.

The oesophagus is the tube food passes down from the throat, through the chest to the stomach.

At the bottom of the chest, it has to pass through a hole in the diaphragm, breathing muscle, which is one of the main muscles forming the LOS. This hole is called the "Hiatus".

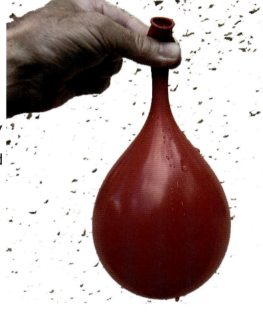

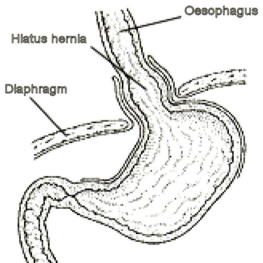

In many people, some of the stomach pushes up through this hole into the chest – a condition known as a hiatus hernia. When this happens, the muscles do not line up properly so reflux is more likely to occur.

Hiatus hernias may develop for many reasons - you can even be born with one, but for most people it is unlikely to cause any problems - apart from perhaps, occasional, mild heartburn which we may treat with an antacid.

Spill concentrated acid on your hand and you'll be scarred for life. The lining of the oesophagus makes mucous to help protect the inner surface but it may not help against a tide of acid reflux and cause scarring and inflammation known as oesophagitis.

Acid will not break down fats and animal tissue so, in the same way as we use detergent to allow water to remove grease from a plate, sometimes some bile is needed to help.

If bile also refluxes into the oesophagus along with the acid, it may start to break down the tissue lining the oesophagus and the body could start to digest itself. For protection, some of the normal cells may be replaced with acid-resistant cells like those found in the intestines. - That's Barrett's.

A paper produced May 2017 [c-iv] suggests:

"In Barrett's esophagus, which can be unambiguously considered as a complication of gastroesophageal reflux disease, reflux symptoms ruining the quality of life may significantly improve, since the metaplastic Barrett epithelium is much more resistant to gastric acid than the normal epithelial lining of the esophagus. Furthermore, the motility disorders (hypertensive lower esophageal sphincter, achalasia, cricopharyngeal achalasia) and structural changes (Schatzki's ring, esophageal stricture, subglottic trachea stenosis), which develop as a complication of reflux may help to prevent aspiration that can cause new complaints and may lead to further complications."

In some respects, Barrett's may be thought of as a slightly untrustworthy friend protecting our bodies from digesting themselves but if you continue throwing concentrated acid over him, he may rebel and have a breakdown so we need to keep an eye on him every few years to make sure he's behaving himself.

Oesophageal Cancer

There are two types of cancer of the oesophagus; Squamous Cell Carcinoma (SCC) and Oesophageal Adenocarcinoma (OAC).
Squamous Cell Carcinomas are more prevalent in Asian countries whilst Oesophageal Adenocarcinomas are more prevalent in UK, Europe and America.
SCC is more likely to be found in the upper oesophagus and is heavily linked to drinking and smoking. Rates of SCC are remaining static.
OAC is more likely to be found in the lower oesophagus and is heavily linked to acid reflux and Barrett's Oesophagus. Rates of OAC are rising rapidly.
In UK, OAC is the 13th most commonly identified cancer, more common in men in whom it's the 8th most common cancer.
Deaths from oesophageal cancer in UK, however, are disproportionately higher with it being the fifth most common cancer killer amongst men and 7th amongst women accounting for one person an hour on average with mortality rates having increased by 65% in the last 40 years.
Treatment for Oesophageal cancer depends upon its stage at discovery.

Staging of Oesophageal Cancer.

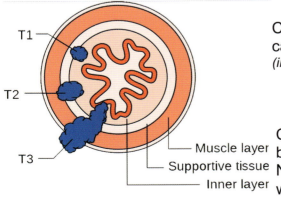

Cross section diagram of the Oesophagus showing cancer stages T1, T2, T3
(image courtesy of Cancer Research UK)

Cancers are staged using TNM codes as described below. T refers to the stage of the primary Tumour, N refers to Lymph Nodes and M to metastasis (i.e. whether it has spread to other organs).

Primary Tumour (T)

TX	Primary tumour cannot be assessed
T0	No evidence of primary tumour
Tis	High Grade Dysplasia ("Tumour in situ")
T1	Tumour has grown no further than the layer of supportive tissue
T1a	Tumour invades the lamina propria or muscularis mucosae (i.e. upper layers)
T1b	Tumour invades submucosa (i.e. lower layers)
T2	Tumour has grown into the muscle layer of the wall of the oesophagus
T3	Tumour has grown into the membrane covering the outside of the oesophagus
T4	Tumour invades adjacent structures
T4a	Cancer has grown into the tissue covering the lungs (pleura), the outer covering of the heart (pericardium), or the muscle at the bottom of the rib cage (diaphragm)
T4b	Cancer has spread into other nearby structures such as the windpipe (trachea), a spinal bone (vertebra) or a major blood vessel (the aorta)

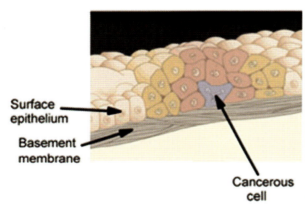

Carcinoma in situ / High Grade Dysplasia

("High grade dysplasia" includes all non-invasive neoplastic epithelia that was formerly called "carcinoma in situ", a diagnosis that is no longer used for columnar mucosae in the gastrointestinal tract.)

N.B. Carcinoma in Situ is not cancer but has a high risk of becoming cancerous.

Regional Lymph Nodes (N)

NX	Regional lymph nodes cannot be assessed
N0	No cancer cells in nearby lymph nodes
N1	Cancer cells in 1-2 nearby lymph nodes
N2	Cancer cells in 3-6 nearby lymph nodes
N3	Cancer cells in more than 7 lymph nodes

Distant metastasis (M)

M0	No cancer in other parts of the body
M1	Cancer has spread to other areas

Dysphagia

Swallowing difficulties (dysphagia) may be attributable to a number of causes. Anyone experiencing swallowing difficulty should see their doctor to have it checked out straight away.

They may be caused by diseases which cause malfunctions in the brain such as Parkinson's, Multiple Sclerosis or Motor Neurone Disease, muscle dysfunction caused by stroke, achalasia whereby the Lower Oesophageal Sphincter doesn't relax sufficiently or stricture or narrowing of the oesophagus which may be due to a tumour.

Swallowing difficulties are usually diagnosed or investigated by a Barium meal or swallow which entails drinking a mildly radioactive liquid and having its progress checked by means of an X-ray scanner.

Self help

The swallowing process may be assisted by cutting food up small, eating small mouthfuls, chewing well and remaining upright whilst the food bolus traverses the oesophagus. Drinking carbonated water can also assist the swallowing process.

If food remains lodged in the oesophagus for more than about 10 minutes, medical assistance needs to be sought.

Strictures are narrowing of the oesophagus which may be due to many factors. Mostly they are benign and may be due to oesophageal scarring from oesophagitis, a hiatus hernia or dysfunctional lower oesophageal sphincter (achalasia) as described below.

In some cases, strictures can be caused by tumour.

Strictures may be treated by dilation described below or in some cases a stent may be used to hold the oeosphagus open.

Achalasia (or cardiospasm) is a comparatively rare condition whereby the Lower Oesophageal Sphincter may not open properly for food to move into the stomach. We do not know why this develops in some people. It is probably due to damage to nerves in the wall of the oesophagus perhaps caused by a virus in early life.

The various treatment options for achalasia include the following.

Drugs may be prescribed which can relax the muscles. They are usually allowed to dissolve under the tongue half an hour before eating. They relax the pressure on the lower oesophageal sphincter temporarily but are not a long term solution.

Botox (Botulinum toxin) injections delivered endoscopically into the musculature provides sphincter relaxation lasting a few months up to a year.

Dilation of the oesophago-gastric junction to stretch the opening may be achieved using a mercury filled bougie (a rubber cylinder that is inserted blindly to the base of the oesophagus or an endoscopically guided balloon that is then inflated at the optimum point. Whereas stents to keep dilations open are often recommended following dilations elsewhere in the body, they are not recommended at the LOS.

Myotomy is surgery usually performed laparoscopically (ie keyhole surgery) to cut the muscle fibres that fail to retract. This provides a permanent solution but may have complications.

PerOral Endoscopic Myotomy (POEM) is a new technique that is currently being evaluated whereby the surgical procedure is conducted via an endoscope.

Complications of any treatment for achalasia include promotion of acid reflux because of the need to keep the LOS relaxed. Frequently fundoplication is offered at the same time as myotomy. [See chapter on fundoplication.]

Nutcracker Oesophagus

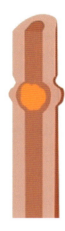

Muscles above the food bolus contract while muscles below relax to help propel the food along the oesophagus.

Many terms are used for **oesophageal spasms**.

"**Nutcracker oesophagus**" usually refers to **hypertensive peristalsis** where the normal muscular action of persitalsis is exaggerated. The oeosphageal muscles contract and relax sequentially as for normal peristalsis but with greater pressure. Symptoms may be hard to define but include various chest pains, regurgitation or dysphagia. The muscular contractions occur as they should but are excessive. When extreme, the condition is termed **hypercontractile oesophagus** or "**jackhammer oesophagus**".

In "**diffuse oesophageal spasm**", the normal contraction and relaxation co-ordinated rhythm of peristalsis is interrupted or out of sequence.

Severity and frequency of symptom occurrence is variable but as it's unlikely to progress to anything further, usually no action is taken apart from pain killers for chest pain. When more severe, it may be treated in much the same way as for achalasia.

Often these conditions will improve over time.

Hypochlorhydria

Hypochlorhydria describes the condition of insufficient hydrochloric acid in the stomach. Whereas acid hyper-secretion is a recognised problem this book talks about, some people have problems from natural hypochlorhydria - producing too little acid. But high dose acid suppressant medication can also result in too little stomach acid - a result of the medicine being too good at its job.

Stomach acid is required to leach essential minerals and vitamins from foods to be better absorbed in the intestines, trigger the production of pepsin and other enzymes and fight unwanted bacteria.

In the stomach, the hydrochloric acid leaches essential minerals and vitamins from foods. To enable their uptake in the duodenum, they are chemically converted to more easily assimilated chlorides.

Hypochlorhydria can result in low vitamin B12 and anaemia through insufficient uptake of iron, hypocalcaemia and exacerbation of osteoporosis through insufficient uptake of calcium, hypomagnesaemia through insufficient uptake of magnesium etc. [c-v]

Another role of stomach acid is to kill unwanted bacteria so hypochlorhydria may result in greater incidence of infections like C-Difficile.

In USA where PPIs have been readily available over the counter for years and widely advertised on television, this has been a problem which led to the FDA issuing warnings against overuse of PPIs. These are powerful drugs whose use should always be monitored by a doctor to ensure they are used properly at the lowest effective dose. Studies have shown "Patients receiving prescription PPI from a GI are more likely to be optimal users with better symptom control. Conversely, consumers are more likely to be suboptimal users with inadequate symptom control." [c-vi]

Hypochlorhydria "side effects", however, have been blown out of proportion. Most patients on minimally effective dose shouldn't experience them. Those taking high dose acid suppressant medication for years, however, should have mineral levels checked by regular blood tests and supplemental minerals may be prescribed. (N.B. prescription of these supplements is required to get the correct dose and formulation. e.g. Calcium Citrate is required to boost calcium levels rather than the cheaper and more readily available calcium carbonate which will only react with remaining stomach acid to lower it further.)

A paper produced in March 2017 [c-vii] provides 10 best practice advice notes including not to take PPI long term for acid reflux alone but that patients with Barrett's Oesophagus *should* remain on PPIs.

Small Intestinal Bacterial, or Fungal, Overgrowth (SIBO/SIFO)
also sometimes referred to as Small Bowel Bacterial Overgrowth Syndrome (SBBOS)

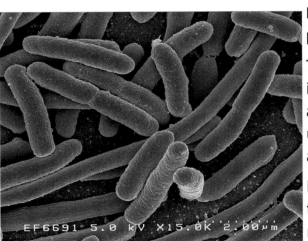

Bacteria abound in the intestines with the predominance in the large intestines.

There are ten times as many micro-organisms in the gut as there are cells in the human body and they have an important job to do in letting us metabolise fatty acids, produce vitamins B and K and far more.

However, with SIBO far more bacteria populate the small intestine than normal including those normally restricted to the large intestine.

(Image of *Escherichia coli*, one of the many species of bacteria present in the human gut, thanks to Wikipedia)

Symptoms of SIBO include those of **Irritable Bowel Syndrome**: constipation, diarrhoea, flatulence, nausea, bloating, abdominal pains and cramps, tiredness and loss of energy (though it is important to realise these symptoms are also commonly found due to other conditions).

The bacteria may rob our bodies of essential nutrients by feeding on them themselves, particularly iron and B12 vitamins which may render us anaemic.

Causes

Causes of overgrowth may not be clear. Some surgical procedures of the intestine and some medical conditions affecting the movement of bacteria down the intestines (the "Migrating Motor Complex") may be to blame.

Another possible cause could be the acid suppressant medication used by acid reflux sufferers. From a meta analyisis published in Clinical Gastroenterology and Hepatology in May 2013, "Proton pump inhibitor use and the risk of small intestinal bacterial overgrowth", the following observation was made, "Use of proton pump inhibitors (PPIs) could predispose individuals to small intestinal bacterial overgrowth (SIBO) by altering the intraluminal environment and bacterial flora. There is controversy regarding the risk of SIBO among PPI users because of conflicting results from prior studies." and the following conclusions were reached, "PPI use statistically was associated with SIBO risk, but only when the diagnosis was made by a highly accurate test (duodenal or jejunal aspirate culture). Differences in study results could arise from the use of different tests to diagnose SIBO." [c-viii]

Treatment

SIBO may be treated with antibiotics but frequently recurs.

There are suggested diets that some sufferers find relief from including Specific Carbohydrate Diet (SCD), the Gut And Psychology Syndrome Diet (GAPS), the Low FODMAP (Fermentable Oligosaccharides, Disaccharides, Monosaccharides and Polyols) diet, the Cedars-Sinai Diet (CSD) and the FAST TRACT diet. These have not been assessed here as are beyond the scope of this book.

Section 7 – Tests and diagnoses

Self Diagnosis

You may be aware of reflux or regurgitation or of the acid burn we refer to as heartburn and this book may make you aware of other possible symptoms you may not have previously considered pertinent. (N.B. Not everyone with acid reflux experiences heartburn.)

It is claimed you can test your stomach acidity by ingesting baking soda and determining how long it is before you belch. Whereas the science behind this has some credibility (baking soda + stomach acid = carbon dioxide = burp), there are so many variables as to make results calculated this way too unreliable for accurate diagnosis.
Other tests of acidity of saliva, urine or blood have no correlation to the acidity of the stomach.

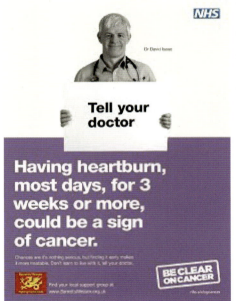

The February 2015 Be Clear On Cancer eosophago-gastric cancers campaign claimed persistent heartburn could be a sign of cancer and to "Tell your doctor"

Action Against Heartburn, the consortium of charities promoting earlier diagnosis of oesophageal cancer, says consult your GP if you have any of these symptoms:

- persistent heartburn (acid reflux, often at night) - ie for three weeks or more
- persistent indigestion, for three weeks or more
- persistent hiccups or an unpleasant taste in your mouth
- difficulty or pain in swallowing food
- unexplained weight loss

Clinical Diagnoses.
There are many tests that may be undertaken to determine whether problems are from excess or too little acid (24 hr pH manometry or Bravo 48 hr ambulatory pH monitoring), swallowing difficulties (barium meal), reflux caused by a weak Lower Oesophageal Sphincter (manometry), Peptest and others but the usual first diagnostic tool is endoscopy when a camera is used to look down your throat and oesophagus for signs of damage or a pill with a camera in may need to be swallowed. It is hoped newer, less invasive techniques (e.g. cytosponge) will be available soon.
Other tests that may be performed include ultrasound, various x-rays and a CT scan.
Results of these tests are analysed to determine exactly what the problems may be so a treatment regimen may be prepared.

Endoscopy

If persistent symptoms of acid reflux or symptoms of concern are presented, the doctor should refer you to a gastro-enterologist who will probably request a gastroscopy. This may also be called an endoscopy or an Oesophago-Gastro-Duodenoscopy (OGD). (Endoscopy refers to probing of any bodily orifices with an endoscope. OGD refers to a scope that looks at the oesophagus, stomach and duodenum.)

What to expect at an endoscopy.

You will usually be able to continue taking any acid suppressant medication. This will ensure your oesophagus has minimal inflammation that may obscure the view.

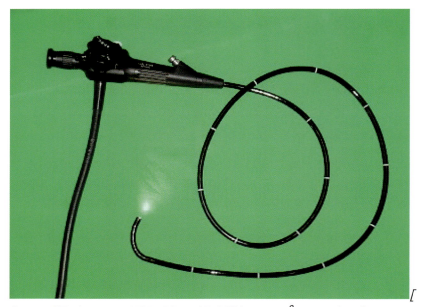

Image "Endoscope, USB, 2015-05-30" by Finn Årup Nielsen]

An endoscopy may be carried out by a gastroenterologist, surgeon or nurse and a few GP surgeries even provide it. It may be carried out at a hospital or treatment centre.

Most patients may opt to have sedation - a drug will be administered by injection that will make you feel drowsy. Although some patients do go to sleep, it is not an anaesthetic but sufficient so you are not aware of the procedure. You will need a friend or partner to escort you. You should not drive or operate machinery for 24 hours afterwards.

Alternatively, you may opt just to have the throat spray to numb the throat but you will be fully conscious throughout and it may not be a particularly pleasant experience. Though you will be OK to drive yourself home afterwards.

Endoscopes have come a long way from the original rigid tubes as thick as a broom handle that were used thanks to British academic Howard Hopkins. Prompted by a dinner party conversation with a fellow medical guest who expressed his frustration at being unable to thoroughly scrutinise the lining of the stomach, Hopkins speculated that thousands of glass fibres arranged in parallel should be able both to shine light round corners and transmit the image back upwards to be viewed by the observer. He spent three years on the project that would result in the fibreoptic endoscope which doctors still routinely use. (Five years later Hopkins would trump this achievement with the laparoscope that would dispense with the need for major surgery for many conditions in favour of the now familiar 'key-hole' operation.)

The long fexible tube about a centimetre in diameter, houses a fibre optic bundle for viewing, one or two other bundles to deliver light and two or three other channels to deliver water and air as required together with a channel for instruments such as snares to be inserted. In addition there are cables to enable the operator to manoeuvre the tip which is flexible enough to be turned to look back at itself.

(The latest endoscopes manage to fit all this into a probe just 5 millimetres wide that can be inserted via the nose if necessary.)

The outside of the tube is marked at regular intervals (usually every 2 centimetres) to enable the endoscopist to make measurements of any suspect areas seen.

You will be given a hospital gown which may usually be donned over your normal clothing.

The back of your throat will be sprayed to numb it. In the treatment room, you will lie on a couch on your left side and a bit will be placed between your teeth that has a hole to permit the flexible shaft of the scope to be inserted.

As the scope reaches the back of your throat you may be told to swallow though this is likely to be an automatic response. Air will be pumped into the esophagus and stomach so the probe has more room to operate without damaging the lining.

The endoscopist guides the scope using hand controls whilst he looks at a monitor usually behind you. If anything requires further investigation (eg suspected Barrett's cells), he'll pass a wire snare down the instrument channel to take a biopsy - a small tissue sample. This is a painless procedure; most people are unaware it has been done. (See the page on Biopsies.)

Typically, the throat, oesophagus, stomach and duodenum will be examined this way.

Biopsies

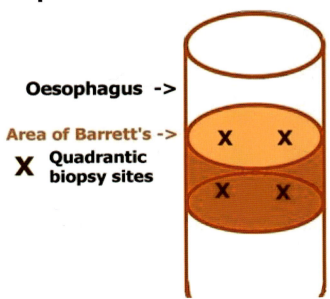

To identify Barrett's and look for possible dysplasia, samples of cells (biopsies) need to be taken and examined by microscope.

The "Seattle Protocol", introduced about 20 years ago, calls for biopsies to be taken quadrantically over each centimetre length of the suspected area.

And it's sometimes not that easy to tell exactly where the suspected Barrett's begins and ends - and it's unlikely to be a tidy ring as in this picture - far more likely to have tongues or islets and the surface of the oesophagus isn't nice and smooth.

The Seattle protocol has come in for discussion with research papers appearing to contradict each other [t-i][t-ii].

A good endoscopist may be able to spot the suspect areas but it can be like looking for a needle in a haystack.

(How quickly can you spot the odd one out?)

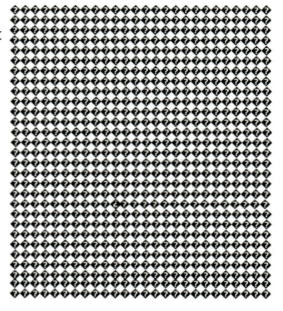

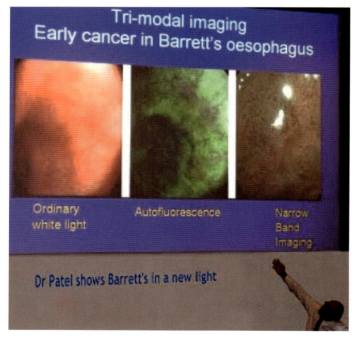

Attempting to make the identification of suspect cells easier, various techniques have been used including spraying the oesophagus with vinegar which makes areas of Barrett's show up better.

Other techniques involve using different coloured lighting; tri-modal imaging utilises auto flouresence and narrow band imaging techniques in combination with ordinary white light. And new endoscopes are now available with in-built microscope functions.

The mined biopsies, each the size of a grain of rice, are placed in a fixative to preserve them and sent to the pathology laboratories where they are embedded in paraffin wax. When set, this is then sliced very thinly to create microscope slides to be examined by a skilled histopathologist looking at the structure of the cells. The presence of columnar, "goblet" cells is indicative of Barrett's Oesophagus.

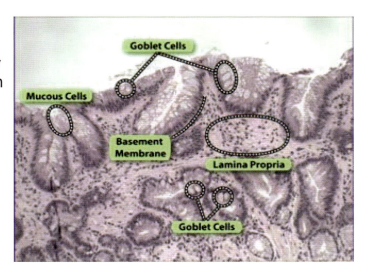

The image on the right shows a typical microscope slide (annotated) where Barrett's cells have been discovered.

The pathologist must also determine whether the cells have started on a course which could lead to cancer, "dysplasia". (See the page on Barrett's Oesophagus.)

Cytosponge

Diagnosis of Barrett's Oesophagus currently requires an endoscopist pushing an endoscope down your throat and taking biopsies from suspect areas to be examined by a histopathologist in the lab. All rather time consuming and expensive (at £600 a time for the NHS).

So doctors are often reticent about referring patients reporting heartburn which is common and usually curable with an antacid or acid suppressant medicine. This may mean patients with pre-cancerous Barrett's may be missed.

Is there an easier (and cheaper) way?

In China, 40 years ago, wanting to see what was going on inside patients complaining of reflux and swallowing problems, a technique was attempted which involved a patient swallowing something the size of a golf ball and regurgitating it. Hardly surprising it didn't catch on, particularly as once regurgitated, doctors had no idea how to interpret whatever was brought up with it.

However in recent years the idea has been reinvented. Squash a sponge ball into a soluble capsule small enough to be swallowed and fastened to a length of string and you have Cytosponge™. The capsule can be swallowed like a tablet whilst keeping hold of the string. The capsule dissolves, the sponge expands and it is pulled back out by the string.

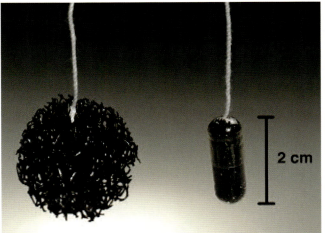

Development of the Cytosponge has been carried out by the Cambridge based team led by Dr Rebecca Fitzgerald and funded by Cancer Research UK and the Medical Research Council.

The expanded sponge and to its right the capsule.

Millions of cells are harvested this way from anywhere between the stomach and the mouth. It is not feasible to start examining them under a microscope as with a normal biopsy so the cells need to be examined in another way.

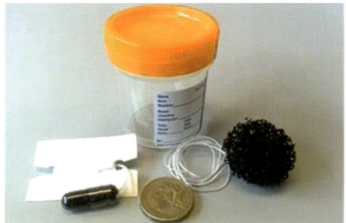

The cells are removed by soaking the sponge in a histological fixative and centrifuging the resultant mass. They are then assessed using a variety of techniques including flowing past a laser in a flow cytometer that identifies cells by the way they scatter the light and looks for specific biomarkers. Biomarkers have been identified that indicate a particular possibility of Barrett's Oesophagus and for Oesophageal cancers.

The complete test kit

If these biomarkers are detected, the patient will require a normal endoscopy for further appraisal.

The advantages of Cytosponge are it is considerably cheaper than an endoscopy (about £25 a time), takes less time, requires less skill (a nurse at a GP practice could administer it) and it could be used as an initial screening for any patient who reports persistent heartburn so more cases of Barrett's may be discovered before it's too late.

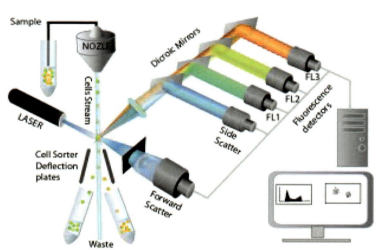

Flow cytometry is one of the processes used.

Peptest

Apart from acid, digestive enzymes are produced by the stomach to assist the breakdown of the received food. The role of these enzymes, Pepsin, Chymotrypsin and Trypsin is to break down the proteins into peptides and amino acids for easy absorption in the intestines.

The Peptest devised by Professor Dettmar, tests the saliva for pepsin. Since this enzyme is not meant to exist outside the stomach, if found in the saliva, it proves the presence of extra-oesophageal reflux. It is an easy test and can even be done by purchasing a test kit for home use.

It has been used to detect extra-oesophageal reflux in children with "glue ear" (otitis media). A paper published in May 2015, "Diagnosis of extraesophageal reflux in children with chronic otitis media with effusion" using Peptest, published in the International Journal of Pediatric Otorhinolaryngology [t-iii] found "Pepsin was detected in 1/3 of middle ear specimens of patients with OME. These patients probably suffer from more severe reflux and therefore would be potential candidates for antireflux therapy. However, this has to be confirmed in further studies."

24 hour pH manometry test

The testing measures the pressures at the lower oesophageal sphincter and your acid levels over a 24 hour period.

You will usually be off medication for a few days before and during the test.

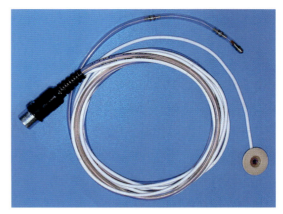
Above: The pH probe

The initial test takes about 20 minutes. A thin tube is passed through the nose and down the oesophagus via the back of the throat. This will measure pressure changes as you swallow small amounts of water, about a teaspoonful at a time, fed to you by the nurse running the test.

The tube is then removed and replaced by a wire with a sensor to measure acidity.

The wire protruding from the nose is connected to a recording device about the size of a personal CD player that is worn on a belt around the waist.

The recorder has three buttons. One is pressed to signal when you start and stop eating, one is pressed to signal when you lie down or stand up and the third is the "event" button to be pressed whenever you experience acid reflux.

The next day, the device will be removed and a print out of the data recorded will show your levels of acid during the 24 hours use.

48 Hour Bravo monitor

The Bravo capsule essentially does the same job. Using an endoscope, it is attached to the wall of the lower oesophagus and transmits the data to the recorder using a radio signal rather than requiring the wire protruding from the nose. It is usually used over a 48 hour period. The recorder is returned to the hospital while the capsule breaks free and passes out through the digestive system within a few days.

DeMeester score

From the data collected, these factors are recorded: the percentage of time your stomach pH is less than 4 (i.e. high acid), the percentage of time pH is less than 4 when you are upright, the amount of time your pH is less than 4 when you are lying down, the number of reflux episodes experienced, the number of episodes greater than 5 minutes and the length of time of the longest reflux incident. From these data a Composite pH score is calculated known as the DeMeester score. Anything greater than 14.72 indicates reflux problems.

Barium Swallow

Doctors can observe how we swallow food by performing a **Barium Swallow** test.

A drink containing Barium Sulphate is administered. It blocks the passage of x-rays which can make its progress through the body visible. Standing in front of an X-ray scanner, you drink the liquid and the scanner watches its progress through the oesophagus. Normal transit would be about 5 seconds but if there is poor peristalsis or nutcracker oesophagus, the liquid may take longer or even flow backwards at some stage. A Barium Swallow will also reveal existence of any oesophageal pouches where the liquid pools.

A Barium Meal is administered to look at the efficiency of the stomach to empty. It is administered lying down with the X-ray scanner monitoring the stomach.

In a recent paper published in Gastroenterology and Endoscopy news in September 2015, researchers at Nottingham University Hospital question the necessity of performing a Barium test declaring an endoscopy to be a better diagnostic procedure whereby detection of cancer (if present) could be dealt with immediately. [t-iv]

The Heidelberg Test

To test for hypochlorhydria or hyperchlorhydria (too little or too much acid), the Heidelberg Test uses a capsule containing a pH meter that is swallowed.

The capsule is usually tethered by a thread so it may be held in the stomach while you are fed sodium bicarbonate to see how quickly the stomach produces acid to compensate.

The test capsule can also help determine the effectiveness of the pyloric sphincter and peristalsis and diagnose gastroparesis (delayed stomach emptying) and dumping syndrome (rapid stomach emptying).

A similar test using an untethered capsule can be used to record acidity in the duodenum and intestines generally.

This is not the same as the camera capsule that may be swallowed to examine the whole gastrointestinal tract nor the tethered camera capsule that may be used to visually examine the oesophagus.

Section 8 – Treatments

Recommendations

These pages deal with the treatment of the possible consequential problems from acid and bile reflux, Barrett's Oesophagus and Oesophageal Adenocarcinoma (cancer).

For treatments to prevent reflux see the chapter on Reflux reduction techniques - medication, surgery and devices.

Because the risks of progression to cancer of "normal", non-dysplastic, Barrett's are very small (see the page on Barrett's Oesophagus), the best advice is usually to leave it as it is but to receive regular surveillance every few years.

Guidelines issued in 2013 by the British Society for Gastroenterology [tr-i], included this map for surveillance of non-dysplastic Barrett's:

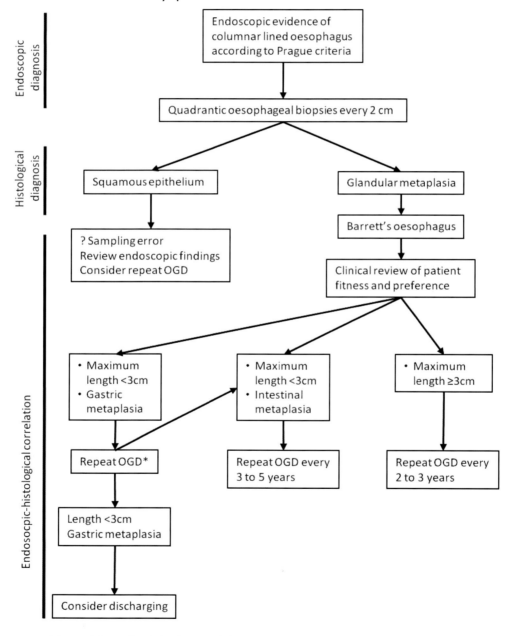

* Interval depends on the degree of clinical confidence about diagnosis (accuracy of endoscopic report and number of biopsies)

"Columnar lined oesophagus" indicates the cellular changes we know as Barrett's.
"OGD" (= Oesophago-Gastro-Duodenoscopy) is the term for the type of surveillance

endoscopy used looking at the oesophagus, stomach and duodenum.

"Squamous epithelium" is the normal lining of the oesophagus.

"Glandular metaplasia" indicates a change in cell structure = Barrett's Oesophagus.

"Gastric metaplasia" indicates the changed cells resemble those found in the stomach.

"Intestinal metaplasia" indicates the changed cells resemble those found in the intestines.

If short segment Barrett's is identified (i.e. less than 3 cm in length), it is recommended surveillance scoping be carried out every 3 to 5 years.

For segments of 3 cm or longer, a surveillance interval of 2 to 3 years is recommended.

However, there is a growing number of gastroenterologists who question the value of regular surveillance, since for the vast majority of those with non-dysplastic Barrett's it will never progress, suggesting it better to attempt to identify those particularly at risk of progression to receive endoscopy.

If, however, dysplasia is discovered, the following map for surveillance is shown in the 2017 revised guidelines [tr-ii]:

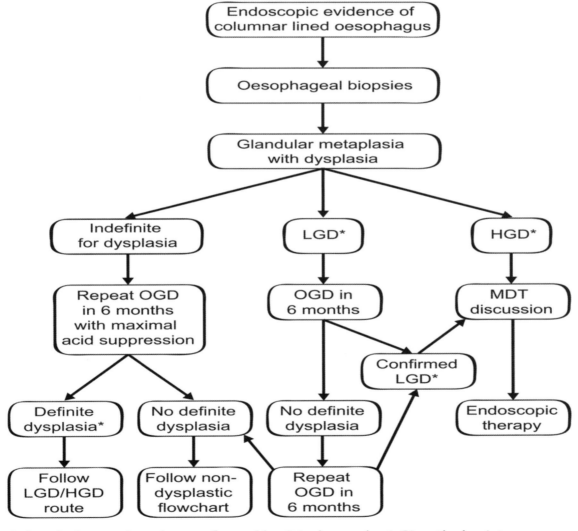

* dysplasia needs to be confirmed by 2 independent GI pathologists

"LGD" = Low Grade Dysplasia, "HGD" = High Grade Dysplasia

"MDT" = Multi-Disciplinary Team Who will discuss treatment options.

"Therapeutic Intervention" may include any of the procedures described on the following pages.

Procedures

Theses pages describe the various procedures that may be used in the removal of dysplastic cells and prevent progression of oesophageal cancer. In some cases. they may also be applicable to early stages of oesophageal cancer.

Endoscopic Mucosal Resection

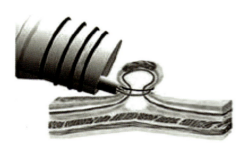

EMR is a technique whereby a small area of cells is removed using a wire snare passed through the endoscope.

The endoscopist identifies a suspect area (usually "lumpy") that he sucks into a special cap permitting a rubber band to be placed around it. The heated wire snare is then used to remove the lump which will be sent for analysis at the pathology laboratory.

EMR is frequently used in combination with other ablation techniques, e.g. Radio Frequency Ablation. EMR removes the lumpy bits first and RFA cleans up the smoother areas.

Endoscopic Submucosal Dissection

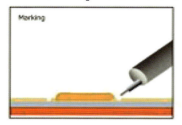 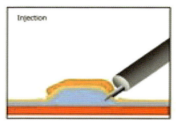 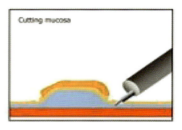
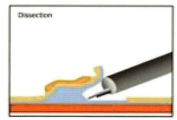 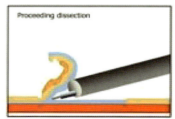 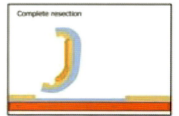

ESD is a recent development from Japan and may be used on early tumours that have not entered the muscle layer.

The perimeter of the lesion to be removed is marked. A suitable fluid is next injected into the submucosal layer to separate and raise the lesion which is then cut away using fine knives via the endoscope.

ESD can remove larger areas than EMR.

Radio Frequency Ablation

RFA is still sometimes referred to as Halo therapy (though that name is trademarked by another company).

Barrx™ RFA is applied during an endoscopy procedure to destroy the abnormal Barrett's oesophagus lining. The lining which regrows is usually normal.

There are two different types of Barrx RFA device. The Barrx 360 device treats the entire wall of the gullet. The Barrx 90 device is similar, but treats a smaller area.

Patients are usually treated with the Barrx 360 device initially and if, at the next endoscopy, there is any abnormal Barrett's oesophagus lining left, retreatment with either the Barrx 360 or Barrx 90 device, depending on how big the area needing treatment is.

During the Procedure

Using standard endoscopy techniques, the physician activates and controls the different functions of the Barrx 360 System.

Ablation

1. The Barrx 360+ Ablation Catheter has a balloon at the tip covered by a band of radio frequency electrodes.

2. Once the electrodes of the balloon are positioned on the desired treatment area the balloon is inflated and a short burst of energy delivered.

    - The design of this technology limits the energy delivery to a depth clinically proven to remove the diseased tissue while reducing the risk of injury to the deeper and healthy tissue layers.

    - The Barrx 360+ Ablation Catheter ablates a 3cm circumferential segment of Barrett's tissue within the oesophagus

3. For patients with Barrett's Oesophagus lesions longer than 3cm, the Barrx 360+ Ablation Catheter is simply repositioned and the ablation steps are repeated.

A report in New England Journal of Medicine in May 2009 concluded, "In patients with dysplastic Barrett's esophagus, radiofrequency ablation was associated with a high rate of complete eradication of both dysplasia and intestinal metaplasia and a reduced risk of disease progression." [tr-ii]

A July 2015 report ,"Comparing outcome of radiofrequency ablation in Barrett's with high grade dysplasia and intramucosal carcinoma: a prospective multicenter UK registry" [tr-iii] concluded, "The Registry reports on endoscopic therapy for Barrett's neoplasia, representing real-life outcomes. Patients with IMC were more likely to have visible lesions requiring initial EMR than those with HGD, and may carry a higher risk of cancer progression in the medium term." affirming the efficacy of combination of the two modalities.

Cryotherapy

Cryoablation freezes the lesion rather than burning it as in RFA.

A 2011 paper on Cryotherapy for Barrett's Oesophagus and Oesophageal Cancer reported: "Endoscopic spray cryotherapy is a relatively new ablative modality for the treatment of gastrointestinal diseases. Spray cryotherapy rapidly cools tissues by spraying them with either liquid nitrogen or rapidly expanding carbon dioxide gas. Initial, nonrandomized and uncontrolled studies show success rates comparable to other ablative modalities for the treatment of Barrett's esophagus with high-grade dysplasias." [tr-iv]

A 2012 report prepared by the Australian Safety and Efficacy Register of New

Interventional Procedures for the American College of Surgeons in May 2012 found: "The results from these studies suggest that endoscopic spray cryotherapy is effective in treating patients with Barrett's HGD and early esophageal cancer, including those who have failed other forms of treatment, at least in the short-term. Specifically, cryotherapy treatment was associated with a complete eradication of Barrett's HGD in 72-100% of patients. For patients suffering from early stage esophageal cancer, a complete response to cryotherapy treatment was observed in 61-100% of patients." [tr-v]

Photodynamic therapy

This treatment is particularly useful when there is high grade dysplasia but no nodules. Here the changes are often widespread and are difficult to see by endoscopy.

PDT can be used to treat a large area.

This treatment does not aim to completely remove the Barrett's Oesophagus although it sometimes does so.

If you have PDT, you will be given a drug which sensitises you to light. You then have an endoscopy, during which light is shone at the area which needs treatment. The combination of the drug and the light kills the targeted cells.

This treatment takes about 45 minutes. The treatment can be repeated two or three times at an interval of three months if necessary and has been shown to reduce the likelihood of cancer developing by 50 per cent over at least five years.

The treatment, using a drug called Photobarr, is licensed and has been approved by NICE for treating high grade dysplasia in Barrett's Oesophagus.

The drug used will cause your skin to be sensitive to light for up to three months.

Take care to avoid bright sunlight during this time.

A paper published in World Journal of Gastroenterology in November 2013 comparing PDT with RFA, concluded, "In our experience, RFA had higher rate of Complete Remission from Dysplasia without any serious adverse events and was less costly than PDT for endoscopic treatment of Barrett's Dysplasia." [tr-vi]

With the advent of newer ablation methods like RFA, PDT is not so widely utilised nowadays.

Argon plasma coagulation

This technique is mainly used to seal bleeding lesions of the oesophagus.

Argon gas is fed through an endoscope and ionised by the discharge of high energy electricty to seal the blood vessels.

Laser therapy

Intense energy burst using laser via an endoscope may also be used to seal blood vessels.

Multipolar electrocoagulation

Like the two previously mentioned procedures, MPEC can seal blood vessels.

All three of the above procedures may also be used to ablate small distinct areas of Barrett's Oesophagus.

A comparison of the efficacy of MPEC and APC in ablating Barrett's published in Gastrointestinal Endoscopy in 2005 concluded, " Although there were no statistically significant differences, ablation of Barrett's esophagus with pantoprazole and MPEC required numerically fewer treatment sessions, and endoscopic and histologic ablation was achieved in a greater proportion of patients compared with treatment with pantoprazole and APC." [tr-vii]

Oesophagectomy

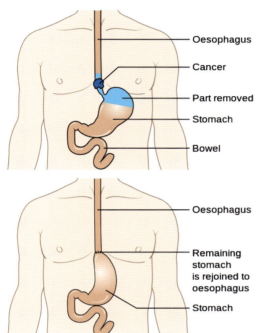

Surgical removal of part or the whole of the oesophagus and or part or whole of the stomach may be performed to remove oesophago-gastric cancers.

The amount removed and the type of surgery offered depends upon the extent and stage of the cancer and the health of the patient.

The diagram shows the typical reconfiguration where just the oesophago-gastric junction has been removed.

[Image thanks to Cancer Research UK]

This type of surgery used to be offered to deal with cases of High Grade Dysplasia to prevent progression to cancer but with the advent of highly effective ablation methods, this is not so common.

There are two ways of accessing the oesophagus to perform the operation: through the chest / thorax (the Transthoracic "Ivor Lewis" approach) or through the abdomen and the hiatus hole, where the oesophagus passes through the diaphragm (the Transhiatal "Kirshner-Nakayama" approach).

The technique used depends upon the extent of the cancer, how much of the oesophagus is to be removed (and whether any of the stomach is also to be removed) and the surgeon's skill and preference.

The Ivor Lewis approach is that most commonly favoured since it provides greater access to the oesophagus but usually requires two major incisions - a midline incision running up from just above the navel and a right thoracotomy incision running around the right shoulder blade resulting in a "shark bite" scar. A technique recently developed by a Southampton surgeon, however, now permits Ivor Lewis surgery to be conducted laparoscopically. [tr-viii]

Depending upon how much has to be removed, the top of the stomach is then typically joined to the throat with the stomach sitting within the chest. For most people, with care, food may be eaten as normal (though in small portions). Some may require foods to be delivered by a J-tube (jejunostomy feeding tube) inserted through the abdomen into the small intestines.

Section 9 – Possible related conditions

Ear, Nose and Throat (ENT)

Ear, Nose and Throat (otorhinolaryngological) problems may be associated with extra-oesophageal reflux. (See the chapter on Reflux to explain the mechanism.) Pulmonary aspiration can take refluxate from the gastroinestinal tract into the lungs.

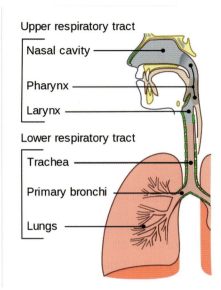

A correlation between cases of asthma and acid reflux has often been observed. "Upper abdominal symptoms, as well as symptoms suggesting rhinitis, were well correlated with asthma symptoms." [o-i]

From a report in Respirology March 2014: "The persistence of chronic cough over time should alert physicians to the possible involvement of GER." and "Until recently, pH-metry was accepted as the gold standard for establishing GER as the cause of respiratory symptoms. But it has now been rendered obsolete by studies ... that confirmed the role of non-acid reflux in patients with chronic cough." [o-ii] putting into question the prescribing of acid suppressant medication to relieve reflux related respiratory symptoms. "Remedial gastric surgery [is] indicated to control severe GER since fundoplication eliminates reflux of any kind."

Though some still advocate that acid suppression may alleviate these symptoms: "Gastro-esophageal reflux disease (GERD) regularly occurs when stomach acid moves up from the stomach into the esophagus. GERD might be associated with chronic asthma symptoms such as coughing and breathlessness. According to several studies on children and adults, GERD is proven to have a close relationship with asthma. Medication treatment via proton-pump inhibitors (PPIs), such as Omeprazole, H2 receptor blockers (Ranitidine), and other antireflux medications, is appropriate for ameliorating GERD and asthma. Moreover, surgery is another useful approach to GERD and asthma treatment. In this regard, Nissen fundoplication (laparoscopic) is a principal surgery method. Medical and surgical antireflux therapies are recognized as effective methods in the treatment of GERD-associated asthma. Our review included studies that evaluated treatment of GERD-associated asthma. These studies accentuated the critical role of acid reflux suppression in relieving the patients suffering from a difficult to control asthma." [o-iii]

Of course, respiratory symptoms may have various causes; reflux is just one of them.

Pneumonia

The symptoms of pneumonia may include:
- Fever, sweating and shaking chills
- Cough, which may produce phlegm
- Chest pain when you breathe or cough
- Shortness of breath
- Fatigue
- Nausea, vomiting or diarrhoea

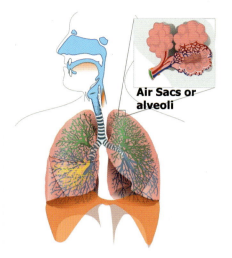

Pneumonia is most usually associated with bacterial or viral infection but may be caused by inhalation of refluxate from the stomach. This is known as aspiration pneumonia.

Pneumonia is an inflammatory condition of the lungs primarily affecting the air sacs (alveoli).

Aspiration pneumonia usually infects the upper back part (posterior apex) of the lower lobe of the right lung though if lying down it can also infect the back of the upper lobes as well.

Pneumonia is usually treated with antibiotics but for chronic aspiration pneumonia, other treatments may also be considered including intubation (insertion of a tube into the airways) and physiotherapy which may include being taught Active Cycle of Breathing Technique (ACBT) to help clear the lungs.

COPD (Chronic Obstructive Pulmonary Disease) and asthma

Damage to the airways from particles in the air (eg smoke) or aspirated from reflux, can cause a narrowing of the bronchioles or blocking from mucous making exhaling difficult.

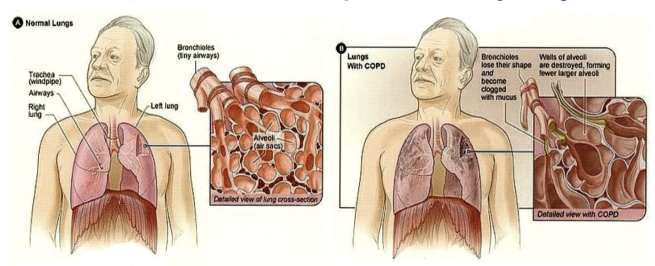

On the left is a diagram of the lungs and airways with an inset showing a detailed cross-section of normal bronchioles and alveoli. On the right are lungs damaged by COPD with an inset showing a cross-section of damaged bronchioles and alveoli.

Bronchiectasis

Bronchiectasis, a permanent dilation (enlargement) of the airways, can be caused by many different factors including asthma, pneumonia and pulmonary aspiration of refluxate from the gastrointestinal tract.

The damaged airways are found towards the bottom of the lungs and are characterised by thickened walls and production of excess mucous.

Symptoms may include excess mucous, cough, frequent chest infections, shortness of breath and coughing up blood.

Crackling sounds may be heard on breathing with low pitched snoring or wheezing.

Since the damage is permanent, treatment is directed at preventing further damage which can include antibiotics and physiotherapy including ACBT as mentioned for Pneumonia treatment above.

Pulmonary Fibrosis

Also called Idiopathic Pulmonary Fibrosis (IPF) when the actual cause is unknown, the permanent scarring damaging the airways may be caused by irritants aspirated into the lungs from airborne particles (eg smoke) or refluxed from the oesophagus.

Figure A shows the location of the lungs and airways in the body. The inset image shows a detail of the lung's airways and air sacs in cross-section.

Figure B shows fibrosis (scarring) in the lungs. The inset image shows a detailed view of the fibrosis and how it damages the airways and air sacs

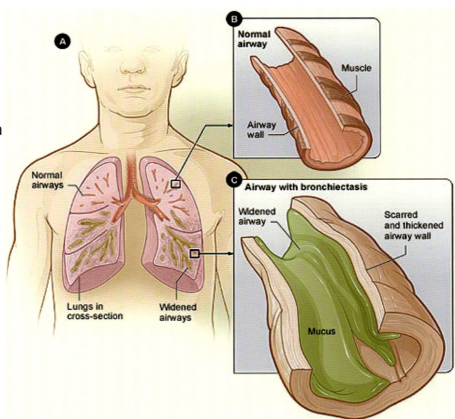

Gastric Dumping Syndrome

Gastric Dumping Syndrome most frequently occurs when a patient has had surgery that has resulted in a smaller stomach. (e.g. oesophagectomy, gastric or bariatric surgery).

With a smaller stomach, it can feel full quicker and dump the contents too quickly into the duodenum by osmosis occasioned by the intestinal contents having more sugars than the stomach contents resulting in a rapid rush of water from the stomach. This causes tummy rumblings (borborygmi) bloating and nausea. That is known as "early dumping" and typically occurs about 30 minutes after eating. The extra liquid rushing into the intestines can result in watery diarrhoea.

Late dumping typically occurs a couple of hours later and its symptoms can include hyperhydrosis (profuse sweating), dizziness, rapid and hard heartbeat and feeling very weak.

Because of the rapid sugar imbalance, the pancreas may produce an excess of insulin which can cause a hypoglycemic event similar to a diabetic which in extreme cases can lead to coma.

Management of the condition focusses on diet. This list comes from CORE charity. [o-iv]

1. Eat small frequent, regular meals

2. Only drink between meals.

3. Avoid too much sugar and sugary foods. If necessary, you can use artificial sweeteners.

4. Avoid excesses of acidic foods eg. Tomatoes and citrus fruits.

5. Excess fat should be avoided

6. Try not to eat late at night.

7. Avoid food temperature extremes.

8. If you are underweight seek advice from a dietitian regarding energy and protein supplements.

9. Increase foods rich in calcium and Vitamin D.

10. Iron, folic acid and Vitamin B12 supplementation may be necessary.

As for a diabetic, if prone to hypogylcemia, keeping a couple of dextrose tablets available to take at the earliest signs will help.

Eosinophilic Oesophagitis

Whilst not a complication of GORD, Eosinophilic Oesophagitis (EoE), also known as the "asthma of the esophagus", may be frequently misdiagnosed as such.

It is a relatively recently recognised condition leading to inflammation of the oesophagus, not diagnosed before the 1970's.

The symptoms are similar to GORD: Heartburn, chest and upper abdominal pains and swallowing difficulties.

Eosinophils are white blood cells which are not normally found in the oesophagus. They are part of the immune system. Whereas not much is known about the condition, it is probably a result of food allergies. EoE sufferers are frequently found to have other allergy conditions, like eczema, asthma or hay fever.

It is usually diagnosed by a failure of normal treatments for GORD and test for food allergies may be undertaken.

The following foods have been found to cause EoE and may need to be avoided; dairy products, eggs, wheat, seafood, nuts.

There is no medication to cure the condition yet. Currently it may be managed with corticosteroids with their inherent side effects.

A paper released in August 2015 by researchers at the D'Or institute in Rio De Janeiro, found a molecule known as macrophage migration inhibitory factor (MIF) was more prevalent in biopsies of patients with EoE and "the early administration of a drug that blocks the effect of MIF prevented the eosinophils accumulation in the esophagus and the development of esophagitis in treated mice" [o-v]

Section 10 – Myths and Misconceptions

False Profits

The unwary may find compelling looking "evidence" presented by charlatans who claim to have discovered a cure for acid reflux related conditions and try to sell their secret for, typically, $40 to download a pdf file.

One of the main reasons for creating this book was to provide a free factual reference to combat the snake-oil salesmen.

1. **Cures for Acid Reflux/heartburn/GORD**. Frequently these contain the advice to eat a particular brand of apple. There is no secret. We all respond differently to foods and finding foods that work for you is the key. Apples may well work for many, particularly if they replace fatty junk foods or something else that triggered your heartburn.

2. Claims that "**I cured my Barrett's**". The cellular changes that see the squamous lining of the oesophagus replaced with columnar Barrett's cells are not reversible. In some cases it may be possible for dysplasia to regress to non-dysplastic state, though those findings could be the results of different patholgogists' anaylses.

When Barrett's appears to have disappeared, it is probably hidden within the corrugations of the oesophagus or a secondary mucosal layer has grown over it, burying it from view.

Acid and alkaline foods

The stomach is a reservoir of highly concentrated hydrochloric acid that can dissolve metal. The acidity or alkalinity of food mixing with it will make as much difference as pouring a kettle full of hot water into the ocean.

If you have oesophagitis, you may feel discomfort as certain foods pass over it, in the same way as lemon juice would hurt a scratch on the skin but it wouldn't cause scarring.

Alkaline water helps lower acid. - *Wrong.*

The only benefits of alkaline water are to the companies selling it on the misconception it will help neutralise stomach acid. It won't. For those who feel it helps, it's only the placebo effect. It may even have a negative effect on physical health and wellbeing. [m-i]

Milk is good for reflux. - *Wrong.*

Although milk may feel more soothing as it passes through the throat and over any oesophagitis, it contains animal fats and reacts with the acid to make casein plastic. It can result in excess acid being produced and even summon some bile into the stomach.

Spicy foods should be avoided. - *Wrong.*

If this were so, you'd expect the highest incidence of Barrett's Oesophagus and oesophageal cancer on the Indian sub-continent and the far east. Spicy foods may give a burning sensation and irritate areas of inflammation but they usually provide no problem unless they are a particular trigger food for you. Some of the spices, particularly Turmeric (Curcumin) may actually be beneficial.

Barrett's causes pain

Barrett's cells are less sensitive than the squamous cells they have replaced. Barrett's itself is asymptomatic. The pain is due to acid reflux attacking squamous cells away from the Barrett's metaplasia. The Barrett's actually means GORD sufferers are less likely to feel pain.

PPIs cause osteoporosis, anaemia, hypomagnesaemia and C-diffficile

PPIs (Proton Pump Inhibitors) lower production of stomach acid. Low stomach acid (Hypochlorhydria) may result in malabsorption of essential minerals such as calcium, iron, magnesium etc. for people using any acid suppressants in high dose over a long period. This can exacerbate osteoporosis, anaemia, hypomagnesaemia etc.

PPIs should be used at the minimum effective dose. If you are on a high dose for a long period, your doctor can send you for a bone density scan and blood tests. He can prescribe calcium citrate to boost your calcium intake (**N.B. *Not*** Calcium carbonate which would just neutralise the acid.) and other supplemental minerals as required.

Low stomach acid can leave you more susceptible to bacterial infection. Probiotics (eg from live yoghurt cultures) may help supplement your body's immune system.

PPIs cause stomach cancer

"Use of PPIs is associated with an increased incidence of gastric cancer. The most prevalent view is that this arises by confounding rather than because PPIs cause cancer. Most cancers found in patients taking PPIs occur within 1 year of their commencement." [m-ii]

Someone who takes antacids every day is more likely to get cancer of the esophagus.

"People who take antacids frequently are more likely to be diagnosed with esophageal and stomach cancer. However, people who take more antacids usually do so because they have reflux. Reflux predisposes one to Barrett's esophagus, which predisposes one to cancer; this is a more reasonable explanation than that taking antacids causes cancer."
[Dr Keith Roach, Herald Review]

There is a cure for cancer, but big pharma is suppressing it - and other myths about cancer

These myths are all debunked on the Cancer Research UK website [m-iii]

Myth 1: Cancer is a man-made, modern disease

Myth 2: Superfoods prevent cancer

Myth 3: 'Acidic' diets cause cancer

Myth 4: Cancer has a sweet tooth

Myth 5: Cancer is a fungus – and sodium bicarbonate is the cure

Myth 6: There's a miracle cancer cure...

Myth 7: ...And Big Pharma are suppressing it

Myth 8: Cancer treatment kills more than it cures

Myth 9: We've made no progress in fighting cancer

Myth 10: Sharks don't get cancer

Appendices

Summary

Acid + Bile + Reflux over time can cause Barrett's Oesophagus.

Barrett's oesophagus can lead to oesophageal cancer.

Lifestyle and dietary changes may reduce any of the elements.

There are medicines available to reduce acid.

There is surgery available that can reduce reflux.

Many new treatments are becoming available that may or may not prove efficacious in the long term.

Barrett's can be treated to minimise risks of progression to cancer.

Reflux (with or without acid) can cause respiratory and other problems.

Appendix 1

Symptom checker

This is not a definitive list but shows the most commonly reported symptoms. Remember symptoms are not necessarily from acid/reflux. Discuss other possibilities with your doctor.

Symptom	Possibly Acid	Possibly Reflux	Other
Heartburn	Yes	Yes	Check heart
Burping or Belching		Yes	
Gnawing stomach pain	Yes		Many possibilities
Chest pain		Yes	Check heart
Bloating			Many possibilities
Food sticking / swallowing problems			**See a doctor** (see "Achalasia" pg 59)
Throat clearing / excess phlegm		Yes	
Chronic cough		Yes	Check other possibilities
Hoarseness		Yes	
Sour taste / excess saliva in mouth		Yes	
Sleep apnoea / snoring		Yes	
Post nasal drip / sniffing / sinusitis		Yes	
Tooth erosion	Yes	Yes	
Partial deafness / tinnitus / dizziness		Yes	
Asthma / wheezing		Yes	Check other possibilities
Lump in throat feeling (Globus)		Yes	
Bad breath		Yes	
Sore throat		Yes	
Dry Eyes		Yes	
Poor sense of smell		Yes	

Appendix 2

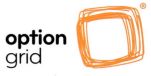

NICE Option Grid for the treatment of long term heartburn.

Treatment of long-term heartburn Use this grid to help you and your healthcare professional talk about the options for treating heartburn that lasts longer than 4 weeks.

Frequently asked questions	Proton pump inhibitor medication (PPI)	Laparoscopic surgery (also known as keyhole surgery)
Why would I be offered this treatment?	If you have long-term heartburn lasting longer than 4 weeks, one possible treatment is to use medication called proton pump inhibitors (PPI).	If treatment with PPI medication is not working or giving you problems, another possible treatment is laparoscopic surgery.
What does this treatment involve?	You take one or more tablets that reduce the amount of stomach acid every day for 4 or 8 weeks, and possibly longer.	The operation makes it more difficult for acidic food to come up into the gullet (oesophagus) from the stomach. It is done under general anaesthetic. It takes a week or so to recover. Medication is not usually needed after surgery.
How long will it take for the treatment to work?	Most people's symptoms improve after a few days of starting this medication.	Most people's sympyoms improve soon after surgery. Swallowing might be uncomfortable for a few weeks, but this goes away.
Will my symptoms get better?	Heartburn symptoms get better in 60 to 90 people in every 100 (60-90%), but symptoms continue or come back in roughly 40 in every 100 people (40%).	Symptoms get better in 90 to 95 patients in every 100 (90-95%). A small number of patients have no improvement.
What are the risks of the treatment?	Risks of serious harm are rare.	As with any surgery, there is a risk of bleeding and infection. General anaesthetic can also be risky for some people. Surgery needs to be repeated in 4 to 6 people out of 100 (4-6%).
What are the side effects of this treatment?	Roughly 7 in 100 of people (7%) have side effects from the medicine. The most common mild side effects are headache, abdominal pain, nausea, diarrhoea, vomiting and increased gas.	Problems after the surgery are common but resolve after a few days. These can include temporary difficulty in swallowing in up to 50 in every 100 people (50%), shoulder pain in roughly 60 in every 100 people (60%), and problems with belching in up to 85 in every 100 people (85%).
How long will it take me to recover from surgery?	Does not apply.	Recovery takes a week or two. Most people are able to go home on the day of the operation.

Editors: Kenneth Rudd, Victoria Thomas, Marie-Anne Durand, Laura Norburn, Toni Tan, John de Caestecker, Mimi McCord, Glyn Elwyn

Appendix 3
Help - where to find more information and get support

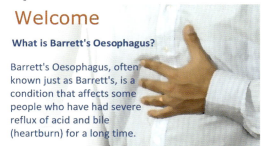

Barrett's UK (Barretts.org.uk) is a directory site for Barrett's specific help in UK including links to all UK charities providing support for Barrett's patients and detailing patient support groups in the UK.

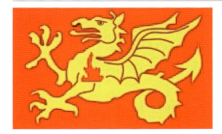

Barrett's Wessex is a regional support charity whose principal aim is *"to reduce the number of deaths to oesophageal cancer through raising awareness of its predominant pre-cancerous lesion, Barrett's Oesophagus in Southampton, Wessex and beyond."*

It has a very informative website at www.BarrettsWessex.org.uk, a Facebook page /BarrettsWessex and a Twitter page @BarrettsWessex and operates the on-line forum, BarrettsCampaign.org.uk/forum

The charity produces a quarterly newsletter, information leaflets and books and holds regular drop-in meetings at venues across the Wessex region together with formal annual meetings open to all.

It offers telephone and text support on 07771 567009 and email support at enquiries@barrettswessex.org.uk

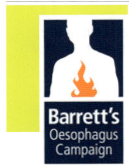

The **Barrett's Oesophagus Campaign** (BOC) is a national charity *"working to prevent cancer of the gullet"*.

It has an informative website at www.BarrettsCampaign.uk, a Facebook page /BarrettsOesophagus and a Twitter page @BOCampaign.

BOC provides leaflets, "What is Barrett's Oesophagus" and "Treatments for Barrett's Oesophagus" downloadable from the Support/downloads page of their website, a telephone helpline and email support at info@barrettscampaign.org.uk

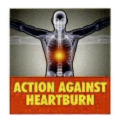

Action Against Heartburn (AAH) is a consortium of the different charities promoting earlier diagnosis of oesophageal (gullet) cancer.

It runs awareness campaigns nationally and locally with the help of its constituent members, most of whom also provide their own support lines:

The Association of Upper GI Surgeons (AUGIS) - promoting establishment of high quality training programmes throughout the UK www.augis.org

Barrett's Oesophagus Campaign (BOC) - maintaining the UK Barrett's Registry, invaluable for researchers www.barrettscampaign.uk

Barrett's Wessex (BW) - the largest support charity for patients with Barrett's Oesophagus - covering Southampton, Wessex and beyond www.barrettswessex.org.uk

Campaign Against Reflux Disease (CARD) - "Tackle Reflux disease early so that you don't have to tackle its complications later!" www.cardcharity.co.uk

Cancer Research UK (CRUK) - pioneering research to bring forward the day when all cancers are cured. www.cancerresearchuk.org

CORE charity - Raising awareness and funding research into gut and liver disease www.corecharity.org.uk

Fighting Oesophageal Reflux Together (FORT) - working closely with experienced local and national clinicians to help patients by providing them with the best up-to-date information www.fortcharity.org.uk

The Gutsy Group - provides support for patients diagnosed with, or recovering from oesophageal cancer www.gutsy-group.org.uk

Heartburn Cancer UK (HCUK) - offering support and information to sufferers of heartburn, Barrett's Oesophagus and cancer of the oesophagus. www.heartburncanceruk.org

The Humberside Oesophageal Support Group (HOSG) - aiming to help anyone with oesophageal problems. www.hosg.org

The Michael Blake Foundation (MBF) - MBF exists to raise awareness of oesophageal cancer. www.michaelblakefoundation.org.uk

OCHRE charity - promoting awareness of oesophageal cancer amongst the public, professionals, politicians and patients www.ochrecharity.org.uk

Oesophageal Patients Association (OPA) - run by experienced patients helping new patients diagnosed with Oesophageal Cancer. www.opa.org.uk

Oesophagoose (National Oesophago-Gastric Cancer Awareness Campaign) - treating patients with oesophageal cancers it has developed an internationally recognised expertise. www.oesophagoose.org

Oxfordshire Oesophageal and Stomach Organisation (OOSO) - providing support for patients across the Oxfordshire region www.ooso.org.uk

The Primary Care Society for Gastroenterology (PCSG) - the voice of primary care gastroenterology that is listened to by those making decisions which affect primary care www.pcsg.org.uk

More details are available on AAH website at www.ActionAgainstHeartburn.org.uk

Appendix 4

The Author's Experience

I must have been about 4 years old when my mother took me to the doctor because I was a "mouth breather" - my nose was constantly blocked. The doctor said I had childhood catarrh and would grow out of it.

It wasn't until 50 years later, I found out it was just one of the many symptoms of the reflux problems I have had to deal with all my life.

All through my life I had problems I now know to have been due to reflux.

I have always had catarrhal problems or rhinitis. I've been tested negative for all known allergens.

When I was six, I had my tonsils and adenoids removed as they thought it would help.

As a boy I had my ears syringed each week - and carry the scars to this day.

I always had a very poor sense of smell and used to get sinusitis and headaches.

I've had my sinuses flushed on a few occasions.

My father ate Rennie like sweets and when I started getting raging heartburn (like a blowtorch down my throat) I did likewise. He died when I was a teenager. It was a heart attack but he probably thought it was indigestion again.

As an adult, I was chastised by my dentist when I had tooth decay accusing me of eating too many sweets.

I have known reflux so bad I have had to sit up for a couple of hours night after night between 2:00 and 4:00am drinking far too much Gaviscon to try and quench the fire.

I have experienced coughing fits, sometimes two or three times a day, where I black out and have had to sit up for a couple of hours night after night between 2:00 and 4:00am coughing and drinking far too much cough suppressant.

More recently I have experienced Gastric dumping Syndrome that may have been the cause of me losing consciousness frighteningly on three occasions.

I have been sent to ENT a few times when I have complained about chronic cough, hoarseness etc. Each time they started by testing my hearing and, when finding it a little deficient (particularly my right ear) have said it may be due to the scarring from all the syringing as a boy. And I have had tinnitus for years.

I was given an asthma inhaler ineffectively.

Suffering from dry eyes, I had a blood test for Sjögren's syndrome but told I was unlikely to have it as I'm a man.

I have experienced achalasia and lying on the ground thumping my chest trying desperately to get the piece of chicken I had just swallowed to move.

I've experienced kidney stones, cholecystitis and pancreatitis. I've had a Nissen fundoplication, cholecystectomy and Collis-Nissen revision surgery.

I spent years on 80 mg omeprazole (and used other PPIs and H2 blockers). I've experienced induced hypochlorhydria: I've been anaemic, unable to walk 50 yards, and may have been hypocalcaemic (fracturing my ankle in a simple fall from my bike).

I have had Barrett's at least 23 years and probably a lot longer.

Following the painful passing of a kidney stone on holiday, the doctor who treated me told me to see my own doctor when I got home. He wanted to know what had caused the stone and on questioning realised it was the excess calcium from all the Rennies. He sent me for a scope. The surgeon brought the screen round so I could see as he pointed out my oesophagitis (which is why I had been taking Rennie), my hiatus hernia that had caused my reflux and the bit that "resembled the intestines" and could possibly lead to cancer. He offered an open operation which sounded horrific and which I declined and started on the recently introduced PPI drugs instead.

It was some years later, with the PPIs becoming less effective and my cough becoming worse that I started researching in the library. When I saw the photos of Barrett's Oesophagus, resembling the intestines and that it could possibly lead to cancer, I recognised it as what I had seen on the screen in that first scope. And I didn't stop researching. And the internet has made that much easier.

I hadn't originally gone to my doctor with my heartburn as I had thought it was normal.

I want to ensure no-one else ignores the symptoms. My Barrett's may never have been discovered. I don't expect my Barrett's will progress but if it did, when would I have found out? When my symptoms were so severe I was forced to, only to then have been diagnosed with cancer too late for it to be treated?

Barrett's Oesophagus is recognisable as a possible precursor to cancer.

Oesophageal cancer is the fifth greatest cancer killer in UK which has the highest rate in the world of this killer that claims the life of one person an hour in Britain on average.

There could be three million with Barrett's in UK but fewer than 10% know it. If those with it can be identified, we may be able to reduce the numbers dying through ignorance.

References

References cited within research papers usually start with the authors' names. Since these may not be readily recognisable to readers of this publication, it has been decided to just provide the titles of papers referred to and the web links to the abstracts of that work where details of the authors, publishing journal and date may be found.

Acid

[a-i] "I have observed that when the use of fat or oily food has been persevered in for some time, there is generally the presence of bile in the gastric fluids." Experiments and Observations on the Gastric Juice, and the Physiology of Digestion by William Beaumont, 1833
Experiments and Observations on the Gastric Juice, and the Physiology of ... - William Beaumont, Alexis St. Martin - Google Books
https://books.google.co.uk/books?id=LOwqAAAAYAAJ&source=gbs_book_other_versions
[a-ii] Dramatic diurnal variation in the concentration of the human trefoil peptide TFF2 in gastric juice -- Semple et al. 48 (5): 648 -- Gut
http://gut.bmj.com/content/48/5/648.short
[a-iii] Host-Bacterial Interactions in Helicobacter pylori Infection - Gastroenterology
http://www.gastrojournal.org/article/S0016-5085(07)02016-1/abstract?
[a-iv] Results - Drug Class Review: Proton Pump Inhibitors - NCBI Bookshelf
http://www.ncbi.nlm.nih.gov/books/NBK47258/
[a-v] Systematic review of PPI and H2A in Reflux oesophagitis
http://www.medicine.ox.ac.uk/bandolier/bandopubs/gordf/gord.html
[a-vi] Esomeprazole provides improved acid control vs. omeprazole In patients with symptoms of gastro-oesophageal reflux disease. - PubMed - NCBI
http://www.ncbi.nlm.nih.gov/pubmed/10886041
[a-vii] Management of reflux esophagitis: does the choice of proton pump inhibitor matter? - PubMed - NCBI
http://www.ncbi.nlm.nih.gov/pubmed/25721889
[a-viii] BMC Gastroenterology | Full text | Gaviscon(R) vs. Omeprazole in symptomatic treatment of moderate gastroesophageal reflux. A direct comparative randomised tria...
http://www.biomedcentral.com/1471-230X/12/18
[a-ix] Proton Pump Inhibitor Usage and the Risk of Myocardial Infarction in the General Population - PLoS one
http://journals.plos.org/plosone/article?id=10.1371/journal.pone.0124653
[a-x] Risk of acute myocardial infarction in patients with gastroesophageal reflux disease: A nationwide population-based study - PLoS one]
http://journals.plos.org/plosone/article?id=10.1371/journal.pone.0173899#sec015
[a-xi] Proton Pump Inhibitor Use and the Risk of Chronic Kidney Disease | Acute Kidney Injury | JAMA Internal Medicine | The JAMA Network
http://jamanetwork.com/journals/jamainternalmedicine/fullarticle/2481157
[a-xii] Proton Pump Inhibitors and Risk of Dementia | Dementia and Cognitive Impairment | JAMA Neurology | The JAMA Network
http://jamanetwork.com/journals/jamaneurology/fullarticle/2487379
[a-xiii] Doctors: Be wary of new PPI studies linking drug to health problems | The Brattleboro Reformer | Brattleboro Breaking News, Sports, Weather, Traffic
http://www.reformer.com/stories/doctors-be-wary-of-new-ppi-studies-linking-drug-to-health-problems,148602
[a-xiv] Proton Pump Inhibitors and Risk of Mild Cognitive Impairment and Dementia - Goldstein - 2017 - Journal of the American Geriatrics Society - Wiley Online Library
http://onlinelibrary.wiley.com/doi/10.1111/jgs.14956/abstract
[a-xv] Proton pump inhibitor use may not prevent high-grade dysplasia and oesophageal adenocarcinoma in Barrett's oesophagus: a nationwide study of 9883 patients - Alimentary Pharmacology & Therapeutics
www.voiceinstituteofnewyork.com/wp-content/uploads/2011/01/PPIs-Dont-Prevent-Cancer.pdf
[a-xvi] Letter: proton pump inhibitor usage still seems to reduce the risk of high-grade dysplasia and/or oesophageal adenocarcinoma in Barrett's oesophagus - Aydin - 2014 - Alimentary Pharmacology & Therapeutics - Wiley Online Library
http://onlinelibrary.wiley.com/doi/10.1111/apt.12892/full
[a-xvii] Proton pump inhibitor use may not prevent high-grade dysplasia and oesophageal adenocarcinoma in Barrett's oesophagus: a nationwide study of 9883 patients - PubMed ...
http://www.ncbi.nlm.nih.gov/pubmed/24617286

[a-xviii] Acid-suppressive medications and risk of oesophageal adenocarcinoma in patients with Barrett's oesophagus: a systematic review and meta-analysis -- Singh et al....
http://gut.bmj.com/content/early/2013/11/12/gutjnl-2013-305997
[a-xix] PPIs Protective for Esophageal Cancer
http://www.gastroendonews.com/ViewArticle.aspx?d=In+the+News&d_id=187&i=April+2014&i_id=1048&a_id=26309
[a-xx] Acid-suppressive medications and risk of oesophageal adenocarcinoma in patients with Barrett's oesophagus: a systematic review and meta-analysis - Gut
https://www.ncbi.nlm.nih.gov/pmc/articles/PMC4199831/
[a-xxi] Proton Pump Inhibitors Display Antitumor Effects in Barrett's Adenocarcinoma Cells - Frontiers in Pharmacology
https://www.ncbi.nlm.nih.gov/pmc/articles/PMC5122752/
[a-xxii] Dyspepsia and gastro-oesophageal reflux disease | 1-recommendations | Guidance and guidelines | NICE
http://www.nice.org.uk/guidance/cg184/chapter/1-recommendations#interventions-for-gastro-oesophageal-reflux-disease-gord-2
[a-xxiii] Is Apple Cider Vinegar Effective for Reducing Heartburn Symptoms Related to Gastroesophageal Reflux Disease? 2015 Thesis
https://repository.asu.edu/attachments/166181/content/Yeh_asu_0010N_15671.pdf
[a-xxiv] Consuming Too Much Apple Cider Vinegar: Here are 5 Side Effects - Foods 4 Better Health
http://www.foods4betterhealth.com/apple-cider-vinegar-side-effects-30850

Bile

[b-i] Chronic diarrhea caused by idiopathic bile acid malabsorption: an explanation at last, Expert Review of Gastroenterology & Hepatology, Informa Healthcare
http://informahealthcare.com/doi/abs/10.1586/egh.09.49
[b-ii] Acute Cholecystitis associated with pancreatic reflux
http://www.ncbi.nlm.nih.gov/pmc/articles/PMC1390992/
[b-iii] American Journal of Gastroenterology - Abstract of article: No association between gallstones and gastroesophageal reflux disease
http://www.nature.com/ajg/journal/v96/n10/abs/ajg2001715a.html

Reflux

[f-i] Heller Myotomy Versus Heller Myotomy With Dor Fundoplication for Achalasia
http://www.ncbi.nlm.nih.gov/pmc/articles/PMC1448931/
[f-ii] Laparoscopic Nissen fundoplication in the treatment of Barrett's esophagus - 10 years of experience.
http://www.ncbi.nlm.nih.gov/pubmed/23837098
[f-iii] 20 years later: laparoscopic fundoplication durability.
http://www.ncbi.nlm.nih.gov/pubmed/25487547
[f-iv] Laparoscopic Nissen-Rossetti fundoplication is effective to control gastro-oesophageal and pharyngeal reflux
http://www.ncbi.nlm.nih.gov/pmc/articles/PMC2639973/
[f-v] Laparoscopic Toupet versus Nissen fundoplication for the treatment of gastroesophageal reflux disease.
http://www.ncbi.nlm.nih.gov/pubmed/14717528
[f-vi] Laparoscopic Nissen Fundoplication
http://emedicine.medscape.com/article/1892517-overview
[r-i] LPR - Aspiration of Upper Oesophageal Reflux (August 2014)
https://sites.google.com/site/robichris/barretts/lpr
[r-ii] Prevalence of Extra-Oesophageal Reflux symptoms amongst acid refluxers and perceived efficacy of regular medication and reflux reduction intervention. (CR 2017)
https://sites.google.com/site/robichris/barretts/prevalence-paper

[r-iii] Nissen fundoplication *vs* proton pump inhibitors for laryngopharyngeal reflux - World Journal of Gastroenterology
https://www.wjgnet.com/1007-9327/full/v23/i19/3546.htm
[r-iv] Heartburn Hell on the NBC Today Show: omitting things consumers might want to know about a $14K device - HealthNewsReview.org
http://www.healthnewsreview.org/2015/03/heartburn-hell-on-the-nbc-today-show-omitting-things-consumers-might-want-to-know-about-a-14k-device/
[r-v] One Hundred Consecutive Patients Treated with Magnetic Sphincter Augmentation for Gastroesophageal Reflux Disease: 6 Years of Clinical Experience from a Single ...
http://www.journalacs.org/article/S1072-7515(13)00356-6/abstract
[r-vi] Device for acid reflux approved by FDA, but not by insurers - StarTribune.com
http://www.startribune.com/device-for-acid-reflux-approved-by-fda-but-not-by-insurers/303946711/
[r-vii] LINX Procedure for GERD: Risks and Benefits
http://www.surgery.usc.edu/uppergi-general/gastroesophagealrefluxdisease-linx-risksbenefits.html
[r-viii] Laparoscopic insertion of a magnetic bead band for gastro-oesophageal reflux disease | Guidance and guidelines | NICE
http://www.nice.org.uk/guidance/ipg431
[r-ix] Removal of the Magnetic Sphincter Augmentation Device: Surgical Technique and Results - Europe PMC
http://europepmc.org/abstract/med/27163959
[r-x] Esophageal Penetration of the Magnetic Sphincter Augmentation Device: History Repeats Itself. - Journal of Laparoendoscopic and Advanced Surgical techniques
https://www.ncbi.nlm.nih.gov/pubmed/28586287
[r-xi] Linx more effective than PPIs for treating regurgitation in GERD - Gastroenterology
http://www.healio.com/gastroenterology/esophagus/news/online/%7B813acc73-b3e6-45e7-926f-103408d88cf2%7D/linx-more-effective-than-ppis-for-treating-regurgitation-in-gerd
[r-xii] Long-term maintenance effect of radiofrequency energy delivery for refractory GERD: a decade later - Springer
http://link.springer.com/article/10.1007%2Fs00464-014-3461-6
[r-xiii] Endoluminal Treatments for Gastroesophageal Reflux Disease (GERD) - A SAGES Guideline
http://www.sages.org/publications/guidelines/endoluminal-treatments-for-gastroesophageal-reflux-disease-gerd/
[r-xiv] Antireflux Transoral Incisionless Fundoplication Using EsophyX: 12-Month Results of a Prospective Multicenter Study - Springer
http://link.springer.com/article/10.1007/s00268-008-9594-9/fulltext.html
[r-xv] Two-year results of a feasibility study on antireflux transoral incisionless fundoplication using EsophyX - Springer
http://link.springer.com/article/10.1007/s00464-009-0384-8/fulltext.html
[r-xvi] Clinical and pH-metric outcomes of transoral esophagogastric fundoplication for the treatment of gastroesophageal reflux disease - Springer
http://link.springer.com/article/10.1007/s00464-010-1497-9/fulltext.html
[r-xvii] EsophyX for Transoral Incisionless Fundoplication (TIF) Proves Itself in Trial (w/video)
http://www.medgadget.com/2013/05/esophyx-for-transoral-incisionless-fundoplication-tif.html
[r-xviii] TIF Underperforming as Long-Term GERD Treatment
http://www.medscape.com/viewarticle/842806?src=wnl_edit_tpal&uac=121783PV
[r-xix] Medigus Announces Completion of First Commercial Procedures in Turkey in GERD Patients Using New Generation of MUSE™ System
http://www.medigus.com/news-events/news/142-medigus-announces-completion-of-first-commercial-procedures-in-turkey-in-gerd-patients-using-new-generation-of-muse-system
[r-xx] First MUSE procedures for GERD performed in Italy
http://www.healio.com/gastroenterology/therapeutics-diagnostics/news/online/%7Ba24031e8-ad19-4194-a529-9e64d20ea82b%7D/first-muse-procedures-for-gerd-performed-in-italy
[r-xxi] Endoscopic anterior fundoplication with the Medigus Ultrasonic Surgical Endostapler (MUSE™) for gastroesophageal reflux disease: 6-month results from a multi-center prospective trial
http://www.ncbi.nlm.nih.gov/pmc/articles/PMC4293474/
[r-xxii] Endoluminal gastroplication for gastro-oesophageal reflux disease | 1-guidance | Guidance and guidelines | NICE

http://www.nice.org.uk/guidance/IPG404/chapter/1-guidance
[r-xxiii] Endocinch therapy for gastro-oesophageal reflux disease: a one year prospective follow up
http://www.ncbi.nlm.nih.gov/pmc/articles/PMC1773510/
[r-xxiv] Long term failure of endoscopic gastroplication (EndoCinch)
http://www.ncbi.nlm.nih.gov/pmc/articles/PMC1774515/
[r-xxv] EndoCinch Procedure: Success Rates
http://www.healthline.com/health/gerd/endocinch-procedure#2
[r-xxvi] StomaphyX Gastric Bypass Revision Surgery
http://bariatric.stopobesityforlife.com/obesity-surgery/correcting-obesity/procedures/stomaphyx/
[r-xxvii] Endoluminal gastroplication for gastro-oesophageal reflux disease
http://www.nice.org.uk/guidance/ipg404
[r-xxviii] Short-term electrical stimulation of the lower esophageal sphincter increases sphincter pressure in patients with gastroesophageal reflux disease
http://onlinelibrary.wiley.com/doi/10.1111/j.1365-2982.2012.01878.x/full
[r-xxix] Electrical stimulation therapy of the lower esophageal sphincter is successful in treating GERD: final results of open-label prospective trial - Springer
http://link.springer.com/article/10.1007/s00464-012-2561-4/fulltext.html
[r-xxx] EndoStim Treats First Patient with Severe Acid Reflux... -- THE HAGUE, Netherlands and ST. LOUIS, Feb. 19, 2013 /PRNewswire/ --
http://www.prnewswire.com/news-releases/endostim-treats-first-patient-with-severe-acid-reflux-in-germany-with-endostim-les-stimulation-system-191921281.html
[r-xxxi] Long-term results of electrical stimulation of the lower esophageal sphincter for the treatment of gastroesophageal reflux disease
https://www.thieme-connect.com/DOI/DOI?10.1055/s-0033-1344213
[r-xxxii] Two-year results of intermittent electrical stimulation of the lower esophageal sphincter treatment of gastroesophageal reflux disease - Surgery
http://www.surgjournal.com/article/S0039-6060(14)00708-9/fulltext
[r-xxxiii] EndoStim Launches Second Generation Neurostimulation Device for GERD -- NIJMEGEN, Netherlands and ST. LOUIS, May 18, 2015 /PRNewswire/ --
http://www.prnewswire.com/news-releases/endostim-launches-second-generation-neurostimulation-device-for-gerd-300084689.html
[r-xxxiv] Electrical stimulation of the lower oesophageal sphincter for treating gastro-oesophageal reflux disease | Guidance and guidelines | NICE
http://www.nice.org.uk/guidance/indevelopment/gid-ip1244
[r-xxxv] Endoscopic implantation of enteryx for treatment of GERD: 12-month results of a prospective, multicenter trial. - PubMed - NCBI
http://www.ncbi.nlm.nih.gov/pubmed/14499767
[r-xxxvi] Enteryx implantation for GERD: expanded multicenter trial results and interim postapproval follow-up to 24 months
http://www.rima.org/web/medline_pdf/GastrointestEndosc_650-8.pdf
[r-xxxvii] Complications involving the mediastinum after injection of Enteryx for GERD - Gastrointestinal Endoscopy
http://www.giejournal.org/article/S0016-5107(04)02645-8/abstract
[r-xxxviii] Public Health Notifications (Medical Devices) > FDA Preliminary Public Health Notification*: Recall of Boston Scientific ENTERYX® Procedure Kits.
http://www.fda.gov/MedicalDevices/Safety/AlertsandNotices/PublicHealthNotifications/ucm064523.htm
[r-xxxix] Visceral artery embolization after endoscopic injection of Enteryx for gastroesophageal reflux disease
http://www.ncbi.nlm.nih.gov/pmc/articles/PMC4242123/
[r-xl] Endoscopic augmentation of the lower oesophageal sphincter using hydrogel implants for the treatment of gastro-oesophageal reflux disease
http://www.nice.org.uk/guidance/IPG222/chapter/1-guidance
[r-xli] A now rarely seen anti-reflux device: The Angelchik prosthesis - International Journal of Case Reports and Images (IJCRI)
http://www.ijcasereportsandimages.com/archive/2013/007-2013-ijcri/015-07-2013-sloane/ijcri-015072013115-sloane-full-text.php

[r-xlii] Dysphagia Secondary to an Angelchik Prosthesis Insertion: the Role of Laparoscopic Management - SAGES Abstract Archives
http://www.sages.org/meetings/annual-meeting/abstracts-archive/dysphagia-secondary-to-an-angelchik-prosthesis-insertion-the-role-of-laparoscopic-management/
[r-xliii] Complications of the Angelchik Antireflux Prosthesis | Annals of Internal Medicine
http://annals.org/article.aspx?articleid=698225
[r-xliv] Efficacy of a Novel "UES Assist Device" in Management of Supraesophageal Complications of Reflux Disease: the Results of a Limited Clinical Trial
http://www.gastrojournal.org/article/S0016-5085(12)60385-0/pdf
[r-xlv] Use of a Sleep Positioning Device Significantly Improves Nocturnal Gastroesophageal Reflux Symptoms
http://medcline.com/wp-content/uploads/2015/04/Gabbard-et-al.-Use-of-a-Sleep-Positioning-Device-Significantly-Improves-Nocturnal-Gastroesophageal-Reflux-Symptoms.pdf
[r-xlvi] A Novel Sleep Assist Device Prevents Gastroesophageal Reflux: A Randomized Controlled Trial
http://medcline.com/wp-content/uploads/2015/04/Person-et-al.-A-Novel-Sleep-Device-Prevents-Gastroesophageal-Reflux.pdf
[r-xlvii] Phase II Trial of Curcumin in Patients with Advanced Pancreatic Cancer
http://clincancerres.aacrjournals.org/content/14/14/4491.full
[r-xlviii] Japanese apricot improves symptoms of gastrointestinal dysmotility associated with gastroesophageal reflux disease.
http://www.ncbi.nlm.nih.gov/pubmed/26185391

Food

[fd-i] No Association of Coffee Consumption with Gastric Ulcer, Duodenal Ulcer, Reflux Esophagitis, and Non-Erosive Reflux Disease: A Cross-Sectional Study of 8,013 Healthy Subjects in Japan
https://www.ncbi.nlm.nih.gov/pmc/articles/PMC3680393/
[fd-ii] Coffee or Tea, Hot or Cold, Are Not Associated With Risk of Barrett's Esophagus - Clinical Gastroenterology and Hepatology
http://www.cghjournal.org/article/S1542-3565%2815%2901616-X/fulltext
[fd-iii] Effects of Alcohol on Barrett's oesophagus
https://docs.google.com/viewer?a=v&pid=sites&srcid=ZGVmYXVsdGRvbWFpbnxiYXJyZXR0c3dlc3NleG5ld3N8Z3g6NDg3YzgzMTUwZDRmYzk4ZQ
[fd-iv] Potential Benefits of pH 8.8 Alkaline Drinking Water as an Adjunct in the Treatment of Reflux DiseaseAnnals of Otology, Rhinology & Laryngology - Jamie A. Koufman, Nikki Johnston, 2012
http://journals.sagepub.com/doi/abs/10.1177/000348941212100702
[fd-v] Alkaline Water Hoax - It is Simple Science
https://www.apswater.com/article.asp?id=198&title=Alkaline_Water_Hoax_-_It_Is_Simple_Science.
[fd-vi] Alkaline Water Helps Neutralize Heartburn Symptoms? Doctors Debunk Claims : SCIENCE : Design & Trend
http://www.designntrend.com/articles/78455/20160613/alkaline-water-helps-neutralize-heartburn-symptoms-doctors-debunk-claims.htm
[fd-vii] The Doctor is In: Water, water everywhere — which drop should we drink?
http://www.tcpalm.com/story/specialty-publications/your-news/martin-county/reader-submitted/2016/11/29/doctor-water-water-everywhere-which-drop-should-we-drink/94591968/
[fd-viii] American Journal of Gastroenterology - Abstract of article: The role of diet and lifestyle measures in the pathogenesis and treatment of gastroesophageal reflux disease
http://www.nature.com/ajg/journal/v95/n10/abs/ajg20001421a.html
[fd-ix] Diet and GERD: Role in Pathogenesis and Management
http://www.medscape.com/viewarticle/875920
[fd-x] Diet and GERD: Role in Pathogenesis and Management
http://www.medscape.com/viewarticle/875920

Complications

[c-i] Barrett's Stem Cells as a Unique and Targetable Entity - Cellular and Molecular Gastroenterology and Hepatology
http://www.cmghjournal.org/article/S2352-345X(17)30079-6/fulltext
[c-ii] UK tops WHO gullet cancer table and obesity may be factor - BBC News
http://www.bbc.co.uk/news/health-29634263
[c-iii] Controversies in Barrett Esophagus - Mayo Clinic Proceedings
http://www.mayoclinicproceedings.org/article/S0025-6196(14)00107-4/fulltext
[c-iv] [Esophageal complications of gastroesophageal reflux disease: consequences or defensive reactions?] - PubMed - NCBI
https://www.ncbi.nlm.nih.gov/pubmed/28502210
[c-v] Long-term Consequences of Chronic Proton Pump Inhibitor Use
http://www.medscape.com/viewarticle/820136_print
[c-vi] Consumer Use of Over-the-Counter PPIs in Patients With GERD
http://www.medscape.com/viewarticle/826831?src=wnl_edit_tpal&uac=121783PV
[c-vii] The Risks and Benefits of Long-term Use of Proton Pump Inhibitors: Expert Review and Best Practice Advice From the American Gastroenterological Association - Gastroenterology
http://www.gastrojournal.org/article/S0016-5085(17)30091-4/fulltext
[c-viii] Proton pump inhibitor use and the risk of small intestinal bacterial overgrowth: a meta-analysis. - PubMed - NCBI
https://www.ncbi.nlm.nih.gov/pubmed/23270866

Tests and diagnosis

[t-i] Systematic Four-Quadrant Biopsy Detects Barrett's Dysplasia
http://www.medscape.com/viewarticle/572642
[t-ii] The Seattle protocol does not more reliably predict the detection of cancer at the time of esophagectomy than a less intensive surveillance protocol. - PubMed -...
http://www.ncbi.nlm.nih.gov/pubmed/19264576
[t-iii] Diagnosis of extraesophageal reflux in children with chronic otitis media with effusion using Peptest.
http://www.ncbi.nlm.nih.gov/pubmed/25736547
[t-iv] Gastroenterology & Endoscopy News - U.K. Study Finds No Need for Diagnostic Barium Test
http://www.gastroendonews.com/ViewArticle.aspx?ses=ogst&d=Endoscopy+Suite&d_id=546&i=September+2015&i_id=1227&a_id=33578

Treatments

[tr-i] New British Society of Gastroenterology (BSG) guidelines for the diagnosis and management of Barrett's oesophagus
http://www.ncbi.nlm.nih.gov/pmc/articles/PMC1856188/
[tr-ii] Revised British Society of Gastroenterology recommendation on the diagnosis and management of Barrett's oesophagus with low-grade dysplasia | Gut
http://gut.bmj.com/content/early/2017/04/07/gutjnl-2017-314135
[tr-iii] Radiofrequency Ablation in Barrett's Esophagus with Dysplasia — NEJM
http://www.nejm.org/doi/full/10.1056/NEJMoa0808145
[tr-iv] Comparing outcome of radiofrequency ablation in Barrett's with high grade dysplasia and intramucosal carcinoma: a prospective multicenter UK registry... - Abstract - Europe PubMed Central
http://europepmc.org/abstract/med/26126159
[tr-v] Cryotherapy for Barrett's esophagus and esophageal cancer. - PubMed - NCBI
http://www.ncbi.nlm.nih.gov/pubmed/21597370
[tr-vi] Horizon Scanning in Surgery: Application to Surgical Education and Practice - Cryotherapy for Esophageal Cancer
https://www.facs.org/~/media/files/education/ceste/cryotherapy%20for%20esophageal%20cancer.ashx

[tr-vii] Photodynamic therapy vs radiofrequency ablation for Barrett's dysplasia: Efficacy, safety and cost-comparison
http://www.ncbi.nlm.nih.gov/pmc/articles/PMC3819546/
[tr-viii] Randomized trial of argon plasma coagulation vs. multipolar electrocoagulation for ablation of Barrett's esophagus.
http://www.ncbi.nlm.nih.gov/pubmed/15729231
[tr-ix] A prospective comparison of totally minimally invasive versus open Ivor Lewis esophagectomy
http://onlinelibrary.wiley.com/doi/10.1111/j.1442-2050.2012.01356.x/abstract

Other

[o-i] The effects of concomitant GERD, dyspepsia, and rhinosinusitis on asthma symptoms
http://www.ncbi.nlm.nih.gov/pmc/articles/PMC4161609/
[o-ii] Gastroesophageal reflux as a cause of chronic cough, severe asthma, and migratory pulmonary infiltrates
http://www.ncbi.nlm.nih.gov/pmc/articles/PMC4184716/#b5
[o-iii] Chronic Asthma and Gastro-Esophageal Reflux Disease: The Treatment Plans
http://jctm.mums.ac.ir/article_4751_0.html
[o-iv] CORE Dumping Syndrome factsheet
http://www.corecharity.org.uk/assets/files/information_pdfs/DumpingSyndrome.pdf
[o-v] Closer to a treatment for the 'asthma of the esophagus' | EurekAlert! Science News
http://www.eurekalert.org/pub_releases/2015-08/difr-cta082815.php

Myths and Misconceptions

[m-i] Negative Effects of Alkaline Water | eHow
http://www.ehow.com/list_7609516_negative-effects-alkaline-water.html
[m-ii] What You Need to Know When You Prescribe a PPI: Cancer
http://www.medscape.com/viewarticle/753221_5
[m-iii] Don't believe the hype – 10 persistent cancer myths debunked - Cancer Research UK - Science blog
http://scienceblog.cancerresearchuk.org/2014/03/24/dont-believe-the-hype-10-persistent-cancer-myths-debunked/

An archive of relevant research links is maintained on Barrett's Wessex website:
https://sites.google.com/site/barrettswessexnews/news/research